# THE ULTIMATE ESSENTIAL OILS GUIDE

## EXPLORE NATURAL SOLUTIONS TO EASE INFLAMMATION, MANAGE STRESS, ENHANCE MUSCLE RECOVERY, BREATHE EASIER, AND ENJOY RESTORATIVE SLEEP

NINA COLLINS

# TABLE OF CONTENTS


*Preface* 7
*Introduction* 9

1. INTRODUCTION TO ESSENTIAL OILS 13
1.1 The History and Origin of Essential Oils 14
1.2 Understanding Essential Oil Extraction and Purity 17
1.3 Common Misconceptions and Myths 19
1.4 Essential Oils vs. Synthetic Alternatives 21

2. SAFETY FIRST: GUIDELINES FOR ESSENTIAL OIL USE 25
2.1 Essential Oil Safety Checklist 26
2.2 Safe Use Around Children and Pets 27
2.3 Recognizing and Avoiding Allergic Reactions 29
2.4 Patch Testing and Dilution Ratios Explained 31

3. ESSENTIAL OILS FOR STRESS RELIEF 35
3.1 Stress Relief Enhancement 36
3.2 Creating a Relaxing Home Atmosphere 38
3.3 Aromatherapy Techniques for Stress Reduction 40
3.4 Personalized Blends for Emotional Balance 42

4. ENHANCING SLEEP QUALITY 47
4.1 Bedtime Routine 48
4.2 Best Oils for Restorative Sleep 50
4.3 Blending Oils for Sleep-Inducing Effects 52
4.4 DIY Pillow Sprays and Sleep Masks 54

5. ESSENTIAL OILS FOR MUSCLE RECOVERY 57
5.1 Post-Workout Recovery Oils 58
5.2 Blending for Inflammation and Soreness 60

5.3 Massage Techniques with Essential Oils 62
5.4 Creating Muscle-Soothing Bath Blends 64

6. BREATHING EASIER WITH ESSENTIAL OILS 69
6.1 Essential Oils for Respiratory Health 70
6.2 DIY Diffuser Blends for Sinus Relief 71
6.3 Steam Inhalation Methods for Congestion 73
6.4 Oils for Seasonal Allergies 75

7. DIY HOUSEHOLD CLEANING 81
7.1 Combatting Bacteria 82
7.2 Freshening the Air: Natural Deodorizers 84
7.3 Essential Oils for Mold and Mildew Prevention 86
7.4 DIY Dish and Laundry Detergents 88

8. PERSONAL CARE AND BEAUTY 91
8.1 Skincare Basics with Essential Oils 92
8.2 Crafting Custom Perfumes and Scents 94
8.3 Hair Care Solutions with Natural Oils 96
8.4 DIY Lip Balms and Body Butter 98

9. KITCHEN AND CULINARY USES 101
9.1 Food-Grade Essential Oils 102
9.2 Flavoring Beverages and Desserts 104
9.3 Infusing Oils into Savory Dishes 106
9.4 Creating Herbal Vinegars and Dressings 108

10. EMOTIONAL AND MENTAL WELL-BEING 111
10.1 Oils for Focus and Concentration 112
10.2 Uplifting Scents for Mood Enhancement 115
10.3 Combating Anxiety and Depression 117
10.4 Using Essential Oils in Meditation Practices 119

11. SEASONAL AND OCCASIONAL USES 123
11.1 Holiday Scents and Festive Blends 124
11.2 Winter Warmth: Comforting Blends 125
11.3 Summer Freshness: Cooling Oils 127
11.4 Essential Oils for Special Occasions and Celebrations 129

12. ADVANCED TECHNIQUES AND LESSER-KNOWN OILS 133
12.1 Creating Aromatic Harmony 134
12.2 Exploring Rare and Exotic Essential Oils 136
12.3 Creating Powerful Oil Combos 139
12.4 Integrating Essential Oils into Holistic Health Practices 141

*Conclusion* 145
*Quick Reference Guide* 149
*Popular Essential Oils* 155
*Essential Oils Terminology* 157
*Success Stories* 161
*References/Sources* 163

*"You are essentially who you create yourself to be, and all that occurs in your life is the result of your own making."*

— STEPHEN RICHARDS

# INTRODUCTION

Amid the relentless rhythm of a vibrant city, Jane was caught in a cycle of deadlines, meetings, and endless tasks. This unyielding pace had begun to leave its mark, manifesting in stress borne of work, sleepless nights filled with unease, and physical discomfort that seemed to echo her fatigue. In a moment of sheer exhaustion, a friend, noticing her plight, introduced Jane to the calming essence of lavender oil. With a mix of skepticism and desperation, Jane decided to give it a try. She placed a few drops of the aromatic oil on her pillow, not daring to hope for much. Yet, to her astonishment, she was soon enveloped in the gentle caress of deep, peaceful sleep—a luxury that had eluded her for far too long. This experience wasn't just a brief respite from her hectic existence; it began an enlightening exploration into the world of essential oils. Jane discovered the extraordinary capacity of these natural concoctions to calm a restless mind, revive a tired physique, and provide comfort to a stressed spirit. Her exploration revealed how nature's offerings could act as soothing allies in the face of modern life's constant challenges.

Whether you're just beginning to explore the potential of essential oils or seeking advanced applications, this guide is your trusted companion. It bridges the gap between novice enthusiasm and expert knowledge, offering a tailored exploration for every experience level. With detailed instructions and accessible information, it accompanies you on your journey to mastering essential oils for enhanced health and well-being.

A comprehensive yet concise guide, it delves deeper than a simple overview while avoiding the exhaustive detail of a lengthy book. This balanced approach provides ample information for thorough understanding, offering detailed insights and practical advice without overwhelming you, ensuring you gain valuable knowledge efficiently and effectively.

As the author of this guide, my dedication extends beyond merely presenting information; it's about facilitating a transformative journey that enables you to navigate health challenges and wholeheartedly embrace wellness. Fueled by a passion for offering guidance that is both dependable and straightforward, I strive to ensure that this book serves as an easily navigable resource for readers of all backgrounds, whether you're new to essential oils or have been incorporating them into your life for years. With an extensive background in the therapeutic use of essential oils, I've cultivated a deep reservoir of knowledge. This expertise is not kept secret; it is openly shared to empower you, the reader, to confidently take control of your health. Through this book, I aim to equip you with a rich understanding of how essential oils work and how they can be integrated into your daily life for improved well-being.

Essential oils are potent, concentrated extracts that encapsulate the essence of a plant's aroma and taste. These natural elixirs have a storied history, tracing their origins back to ancient civilizations like Egypt, India, and China, where they were highly esteemed for their healing and restorative properties. Traditionally, essential oils have been extracted using methods such as steam distillation, a process that involves passing steam through plant material to capture the volatile compounds responsible for the plant's fragrance and therapeutic benefits. In our contemporary lives, essential oils offer a bridge to the wisdom of the past, presenting a holistic approach to wellness that complements modern medicine. They possess the unique ability to soothe the mind, invigorate the senses, and restore balance to the body's systems, thereby providing a multifaceted tool for enhancing our health naturally. Whether used in aromatherapy, topical applications, or as part of daily health routines, essential oils serve as versatile allies in our quest for well-being, embodying the power of nature to nurture and heal.

This guide distinguishes itself with its distinct offerings. Within these pages, you'll discover a wealth of recipes, hands-on uses, and comprehensive safety instructions. These elements ensure a thorough understanding of essential oils and their effective use. Designed to be both informative and practical, this book provides you with the essential tools to succeed.

As you move through the chapters, I encourage you to not just read but actively engage in trying the recipes and applications detailed within. Participate in hands-on experimentation to truly grasp the essence and benefits of each oil. This exploratory process is key to uncovering the unique combinations and methods that resonate most with your personal health and wellness goals. By thoughtfully integrating these oils into your daily routines, you're taking proactive steps toward cultivating a healthier, more vibrant lifestyle.

My goal with this book is to share knowledge and practical tools for a healthier lifestyle using natural remedies. I aim to create an environment that encourages you to improve your health and well-being through essential oils. By the end of this guide, I hope you feel informed and confident in integrating essential oils into your life, fostering positive changes. This comprehensive resource is designed to enhance your physical, mental, emotional, and spiritual wellness, empowering you to find natural solutions for a more fulfilled and harmonious life.

Join me on this journey. Let's explore the wonders of essential oils together and discover how they can transform your well-being. This book is more than a guide; it's an invitation to embrace a natural path to health and happiness.

# 1

# INTRODUCTION TO ESSENTIAL OILS

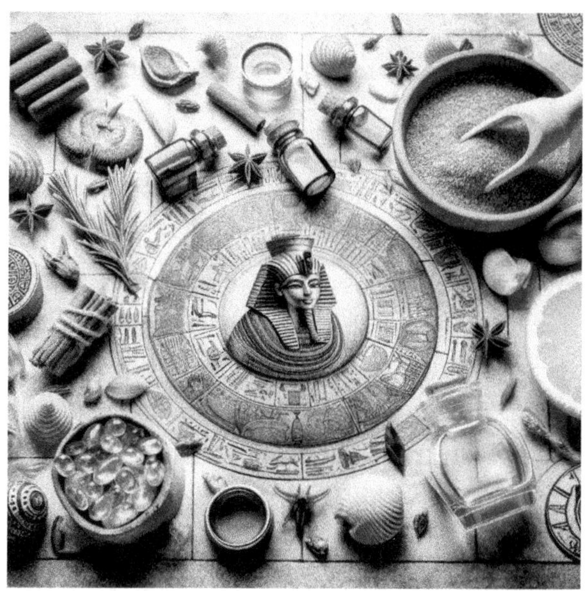

Think back to a time when you sought relief from a headache or needed a moment of calm on a hectic day. You might have reached for a peppermint-infused balm or taken a deep breath of lavender's soothing aroma. Such experiences are not just modern conveniences; they are echoes of ancient practices that have embraced the power of essential oils for thousands of years. This chapter sets the stage for a deep exploration of these remarkable oils, offering the historical backdrop and cultural significance shaping their journey to the present day.

## 1.1 THE HISTORY AND ORIGIN OF ESSENTIAL OILS

Essential oils boast a storied past that stretches across continents and epochs, deeply entrenched in the traditions of the ancients. In the realm of Ancient Egypt, these oils transcended their status as mere luxuries to become staples of everyday life and ceremonial practices. Notably, frankincense and myrrh stood at the forefront of these traditions, serving both to preserve and to protect. It was held that these oils aided in the soul's journey to the afterlife, a testament to their profound aromas and their pivotal role in religious rites, symbolizing holiness and purity. Their value was not confined to the spiritual alone; the Egyptians possessed a profound knowledge of the oils' healing properties. These were woven into their skincare rituals, exploiting their restorative, moisturizing, and rejuvenating effects—qualities especially prized in the unforgiving desert climate. This comprehensive embrace of essential oils illustrates their diverse applications in ancient Egyptian society, meeting both the spiritual and the practical needs of the day.

In the East, traditional Chinese medicine (TCM) has long acknowledged the powerful therapeutic properties of essential oils. TCM practitioners carefully prescribed oils such as ginger and cinnamon not just as remedies but as essential components for balancing the body's energy, known as "qi." They believed these oils were vital for maintaining health and harmony within the body. Revered for their warming and refreshing qualities, these oils were often incorporated into complex herbal formulations aimed at addressing a wide range of ailments. Their use demonstrated a sophisticated understanding of the interconnectedness between nature and human well-being.

Parallel to this, in the heart of India, Ayurveda—considered by many as the world's oldest holistic healing system—has historically placed a profound emphasis on the use of essential oils. Oils derived from sandalwood, holy basil, and a plethora of other plants were not only valued for their aromatic properties but were also believed to hold the power to promote both physical and spiritual well-being. Ayurvedic practices utilize these oils in a range of ways, from direct application in massage and skin care to their inclusion in medicinal concoctions, showcasing a deep-seated belief in their capacity to heal, rejuvenate, and restore balance. This rich tradition of using essential oils in both TCM and Ayurveda highlights a shared understanding across cultures of the intrinsic link between nature's bounty and human health. The enduring use of these ancient systems of medicine underscores the timeless appeal of natural remedies and the wisdom of integrating them into contemporary wellness practices.

As the narrative of essential oils unfolded through the ages, their journey took a pivotal turn upon reaching Europe. It was here during the medieval period that the art of distillation began to emerge, setting the stage for a transformative chapter in their history. The Renaissance era heralded a renaissance of its own in the realm of essential oils. Illustrious figures such as Paracelsus and Avicenna made significant strides in the field, marrying the ancient art of herbalism with the burgeoning field of medicine. Their pioneering work in understanding how essential oils could be distilled and harnessed for their medicinal properties laid the foundational stones for what we recognize today as modern aromatherapy. This period breathed new life into the use of essential oils, melding the era's thirst for scientific discovery with a reverent continuation of age-old healing traditions.

The evolution of essential oils is not just a tale of ancient wisdom but also one of cultural exchange and trade. The Silk Road, a network of trade routes connecting the East and West, was pivotal in distributing these precious oils. Merchants traveled great distances, carrying oils like rose and cedarwood, embedding them into the commerce and culture of new lands. Essential oils also held a place in religious and spiritual ceremonies across different cultures — from anointing rituals in Christianity to purifying practices in Hinduism — underscoring their enduring significance.

The historical uses of essential oils inform their contemporary applications, bridging the gap between ancient traditions and modern wellness practices. Today, we see these oils incorporated into a wide range of products, from skincare to cleaning solutions, each using a nod to the past. The connection between historical practices and current trends reveals a timeless appreciation for the natural healing properties of essential oils. Understanding this history enriches our appreciation and guides us in using these oils conscientiously, ensuring they remain a valuable part of our health and well-being toolkit.

## 1.2 UNDERSTANDING ESSENTIAL OIL EXTRACTION AND PURITY

The journey from plant to bottle is a complex dance of science and nature, with each step in the extraction process playing a crucial role in defining the quality and character of the oils we use. Steam distillation is at the heart of this process, one of the oldest and most common methods. It involves passing steam through plant material and vaporizing the volatile compounds. As the steam rises, it carries these aromatic compounds, condensing into a liquid form. This method is particularly suited to plants like lavender and eucalyptus, where the heat gently coaxes out the oils without altering their chemical integrity excessively. The end product is a pure oil that retains the therapeutic essence of the plant.

On the other hand, cold-press extraction is a method best suited for citrus fruits like oranges and lemons. Here, the technique involves mechanically pressing the peels to release the oils, capturing the vibrant, fresh essence of the citrus without applying heat. This process highlights citrus oils' bright and zesty nature, ensuring their delicate top notes remain intact and untainted by heat-induced degradation. The result is an oil bursting with energy and freshness, perfect for uplifting blends and culinary uses.

Solvent extraction offers a solution for flowers that are too delicate to withstand steam. This method uses solvents like ethanol to gently draw out oils from petals, preserving the fragile aromatic compounds. The solvents are later removed, leaving behind a concentrated essence known as an "absolute," often used in perfumery. This process, though effective, requires precision to ensure no solvent residues remain, maintaining the purity and safety of the oil.

Purity stands as the fundamental pillar of high-quality essential oils, essential for both their effectiveness and safety. It's imperative for consumers to understand the characteristics of pure oil, as this significantly influences its therapeutic benefits and user safety. The pinnacle of purity assessment is Gas Chromatography-Mass Spectrometry (GC/MS) testing, a sophisticated analytical technique that deconstructs the oil into its individual components to detect any adulterants or synthetic substances. Oils that are confirmed to meet the stringent requirements for therapeutic-grade status have undergone extensive testing to guarantee their freedom from any contaminants, ensuring they preserve the entire spectrum of the plant's beneficial compounds. This level of purity is vital for those seeking the full therapeutic potential of essential oils.

The method of extraction also influences an oil's therapeutic benefits. An improperly extracted oil may lose some beneficial properties, reducing its efficacy. For example, excessive heat can degrade delicate compounds, diminishing the oil's potency. This is why choosing the proper extraction method for each plant type is essential to maintaining the oil's integrity and effectiveness.

Sourcing and sustainability are equally vital in the world of essential oils. The demand for these natural products has led to increased scrutiny over how they are harvested.

Wildcrafted oils are sourced from plants growing in their natural habitat, offering a purity and potency that cultivated sources might need to improve. However, this method must be balanced with environmental responsibility, ensuring that harvesting practices do not disrupt local ecosystems or lead to overexploitation. On the other hand, sustainable harvesting practices involve cultivating plants under controlled conditions, often using organic methods to minimize environmental impact. This approach ensures a steady supply of high-quality oils while respecting the planet's natural resources.

Understanding these extraction methods and purity standards empowers you as a consumer. By making informed choices, you can enjoy the full benefits of essential oils while supporting ethical and sustainable practices. This knowledge enhances your wellness and contributes to a more significant movement towards environmental stewardship and responsible consumption.

## 1.3 COMMON MISCONCEPTIONS AND MYTHS

Essential oils have captivated the interest of many, promising a natural approach to health and wellness. However, as with any popular trend, a cloud of misconceptions often hovers, potentially leading people astray. One of the most pervasive myths is the belief that all essential oils are safe for ingestion. While some oils are food-grade and can be used in culinary settings, many are not. Ingesting oils without proper guidance can lead to adverse reactions. For instance, wintergreen oil containing methyl salicylate is toxic if consumed significantly. Understanding each oil's properties and the human body's response is vital. Consulting with a qualified aromatherapist or healthcare provider is essential before considering ingestion.

Another widespread myth suggests that pure essential oils do not expire. This misconception can be misleading and dangerous, as oils degrade over time. Factors such as exposure to light, heat, and air can cause oils to oxidize, losing their potency and potentially becoming irritants. While some oils, like patchouli and sandalwood, improve with age, most do not. Recognizing the signs of expiration, such as changes in aroma or consistency, helps ensure safe use. Proper storage in dark glass bottles, away from direct sunlight and extreme temperatures, can extend an oil's shelf life, but ultimately, awareness of expiration is crucial.

The digital age has amplified the reach of essential oil information, but not all sources are reliable. With online communities brimming with advice, it's vital to distinguish fact from fiction. Misinformation can spread rapidly, and users must exercise caution. To verify information, seek out reputable sources such as certified aromatherapy schools, peer-reviewed studies, and books authored by experts in the field. Avoid relying solely on anecdotal evidence or unverified testimonials. Instead, prioritize evidence-based information that aligns with scientific understanding and established safety guidelines.

Essential oils are respected in holistic health, but their benefits often become exaggerated. It is necessary to differentiate between realistic applications supported by research and overly ambitious ones. For example, studies indicate that lavender oil can aid relaxation and sleep, and tea tree oil has proven antiseptic properties. However, claims that oils can cure serious diseases lack scientific backing. Understanding the scope of what oils can realistically achieve helps users make informed decisions, avoiding disappointment or misuse.

Emphasizing informed and safe use is paramount when discussing essential oils. Users should approach these potent substances with the respect they deserve, appreciating both their power and limitations. This means conducting thorough research and understanding each oil's properties, contraindications, and proper application methods. Safety should always remain a priority, with dilution guidelines followed closely to prevent skin irritation or sensitization. By doing so, one can harness the true potential of essential oils, using them effectively and responsibly to enhance well-being without falling victim to misconceptions or misinformation.

## 1.4 ESSENTIAL OILS VS. SYNTHETIC ALTERNATIVES

When one compares natural essential oils to their synthetic counterparts, the distinction lies in the complexity and authenticity of their composition. Natural oils are complex and nuanced, containing various compounds that work together to create their unique properties and effects. Each drop is a miniature ecosystem, reflecting the intricate balance of a plant's chemistry. These oils are like a symphony, where each component plays its part to produce a harmonious and therapeutic effect. Synthetic oils, however, are often simplified imitations crafted in a lab to mimic the scent of their natural counterparts. While they may capture the aroma, they lack the depth and complexity of natural oils. This simplicity means they often offer different therapeutic benefits, missing the rich array of molecules contributing to an oil's holistic impact.

Choosing natural essential oils over synthetic ones offers several advantages, particularly regarding health and environmental impact. Natural oils are free from artificial additives and potential allergens commonly found in synthetic versions. Synthetic oils, often derived from petrochemicals, can include components that may irritate or cause allergic reactions in sensitive individuals. Additionally, natural oils are biodegradable, breaking down into harmless compounds that do not linger in the environment. Contrast this with synthetic oils, which may contribute to pollution due to their non-biodegradable nature. The use of natural essential oils, therefore, aligns with a commitment to sustainability and ecological responsibility.

There are scenarios where synthetic oils might be appropriate, particularly in industrial contexts where cost-efficiency is paramount. For example, in large-scale manufacturing of household products or perfumes, synthetics offer a consistent and inexpensive alternative produced in bulk. Their uniformity in scent and stability under various conditions makes them suitable for applications where therapeutic benefits are not a priority. However, the preference for natural oils is clear in personal wellness and therapeutic settings. Their holistic value extends beyond fragrance, offering emotional, psychological, and physiological benefits synthetics cannot replicate. Natural oils engage the senses to promote well-being, grounding, and healing, enhancing personal care routines with an authentic touch of nature.

The choice between natural and synthetic reminds us of the broader preference for authenticity over imitation. Using pure essential oils invites the full spectrum of nature's benefits into our lives. These oils are more than just pleasant scents; they serve as tools for enhancing our daily experiences and supporting our health. Whether used in a soothing bath, an invigorating massage, or a calming diffuser blend, natural oils offer a connection to the natural world that synthetics simply cannot. Embracing them in our routines is embracing nature, allowing us to benefit from its wisdom and balance. As we move forward in this exploration, consider the impact of each choice, not only on personal health but also on the collective well-being of our planet. By choosing nature, we choose a path of harmony and respect for the intricate web of life that sustains us.

2

# SAFETY FIRST: GUIDELINES FOR ESSENTIAL OIL USE

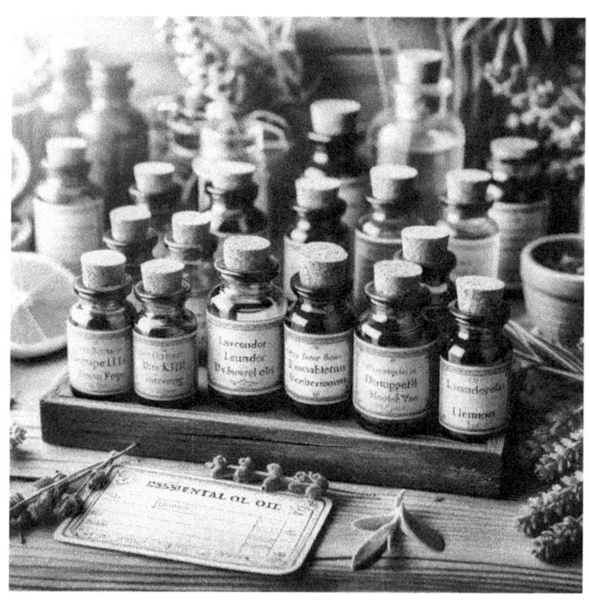

To understand essential oils, it is important to recognize both their benefits and potential risks, including the risk of phototoxicity. Among them, Phototoxicity stands out as a crucial consideration. This phenomenon occurs when certain essential oils, primarily those extracted from citrus fruits, react adversely upon exposure to ultraviolet (UV) light. Once these oils are absorbed, the skin becomes unusually sensitive to sunlight, leading to reactions ranging from mild redness to severe burns. The primary culprits of phototoxicity include oils such as bergamot, lemon, lime, and grapefruit. Not all uses pose a risk; phototoxic reactions typically occur when these oils are applied directly to the skin without dilution and then exposed to sunlight. Following a few guidelines is advisable to safely enjoy the benefits of these vibrant citrus oils while minimizing risks. First, always dilute phototoxic oils before topical application, using a carrier oil to mitigate their concentration.

Moreover, after applying these oils, it's wise to avoid direct sunlight or UV exposure for at least 12 to 24 hours. For sun-safe alternatives, consider using steam-distilled versions of citrus oils, which significantly reduce the risk of phototoxicity, or opt for non-phototoxic citrus oils like sweet orange. Understanding and respecting the potential for phototoxic reactions enables the safe and effective use of essential oils, ensuring that many benefits can be enjoyed without unintended consequences.

## 2.1 ESSENTIAL OIL SAFETY CHECKLIST

1. Read Labels Thoroughly: Pay attention to usage instructions and warnings.
2. Avoid Sensitive Areas: Keep oils away from eyes and mucous membranes.

3. Store Properly: Keep dark glass bottles in a cool, dark place.
4. Watch for Phototoxicity: Be cautious when using citrus oils and sun exposure.
5. Choose Quality: Buy from reputable sources with transparency in testing.

These guidelines form the foundation of safe essential oil use, allowing you to explore their benefits with peace of mind. By respecting these principles, you can fully enjoy the therapeutic potential of essential oils, enhancing your well-being in a responsible and informed manner.

## 2.2 SAFE USE AROUND CHILDREN AND PETS

When it comes to children, the allure of essential oils often lies in their natural origins and soothing properties. However, their concentrated nature requires careful handling, especially with young ones. For infants, the list of safe oils is short. Lavender and chamomile are generally well-tolerated and can provide calming effects, but even these should be used sparingly and always diluted. As children grow, their tolerance to oils increases, allowing for a broader range of oils to be introduced. Dilution is key. A young child's skin is sensitive, so using a higher dilution than you might use for an adult is vital. Typically, a ratio of one drop of essential oil to a tablespoon of carrier oil is a safe starting point. Never apply oils directly on a child's skin without proper dilution, and always do a patch test to check for any reactions.

Like children, pets are family members and deserve the same cautious consideration. While essential oils can offer benefits like calming anxious pets or repelling insects, knowing which oils are safe is crucial. Dogs can generally tolerate oils like lavender and chamomile, which can help soothe their nerves. However, cats are a different story. Their unique metabolism makes them more sensitive, and oils such as tea tree or eucalyptus can be toxic to them. Always avoid using oils directly on your pets. Instead, consider using a diffuser in a well-ventilated area, ensuring your pet can leave the room if they wish. This will allow them to benefit from the oils without direct contact.

Incorporating essential oils into family life requires practical strategies to ensure everyone's safety. For instance, using diffusers in shared living spaces can create a welcoming and calm environment. However, keeping concentration low is important to avoid overwhelming the senses, especially for small children and pets. Always ensure the room is well-ventilated, allowing fresh air to circulate and preventing intense aroma buildup. Avoid applying oils directly to your children's or pets' skin. Instead, add a few drops to a diffuser or mix them into a DIY room spray. This indirect application allows you to enjoy the benefits of oils without the risks associated with direct contact.

Identifying any adverse reactions is crucial for the safe application of essential oils. For children, look out for symptoms of skin irritation, including redness, itching, or swelling, and be vigilant for signs of respiratory distress, such as coughing or wheezing. Should these symptoms manifest, discontinue the oil's use immediately and gently cleanse the area with water and a gentle soap. In pets, recognize signs like excessive drooling, vomiting, or unusual lethargy. In both scenarios, seeking advice from a healthcare provider or veterinarian is advisable without delay. Being aware of these indicators allows for quick action, ensuring the well-being and safety of your loved ones.

Following these safety measures allows you to responsibly integrate essential oils into your household. Essential oils can enhance the atmosphere, creating a serene and supportive space. Remember, a cautious approach allows you to harness the full benefits of essential oils, ensuring a safe environment for every family member.

## 2.3 RECOGNIZING AND AVOIDING ALLERGIC REACTIONS

Imagine applying a new essential oil blend to your wrist, only to find your skin reddening and itching minutes later. This is a classic example of an allergic reaction, where your immune system mistakenly identifies a substance as harmful and overreacts. Despite their natural origins, essential oils contain potent compounds that can trigger such responses. Common symptoms include rashes, hives, and headaches. These reactions occur because the body releases histamines in response to the perceived threat, leading to inflammation and discomfort. Recognizing these signs is the first step in avoiding more severe reactions.

Some oils are notorious for causing allergic reactions more frequently than others. Cinnamon oil, with its spicy warmth, is a prime example. It contains cinnamaldehyde, a compound known to irritate the skin and mucous membranes. Clove oil, another rich and aromatic oil, can also provoke strong reactions due to its high eugenol content, which can cause sensitization. These oils, among others, should be used cautiously, especially if you're prone to allergies. It's wise to research each new oil before using it, checking for common allergens and understanding its chemical profile.

Adopting safe usage practices is crucial to minimize the risk of allergic reactions. Conducting a patch test is a simple yet effective method. Apply a diluted oil mixture to a small patch of skin, like the inside of your forearm, and wait 24 hours to observe any adverse reactions. This test helps identify potential sensitivities before you apply oils more broadly. Gradually introducing new oils into your routine also helps your body adjust and notice subtle changes or reactions. Start with low concentrations and increase if no response occurs. This cautious approach can prevent many uncomfortable situations.

If you experience an adverse reaction, knowing how to respond quickly is essential. First, thoroughly wash the affected area with mild soap and cool water to remove the oil. Avoid hot water, which can open pores and allow more oil to penetrate the skin. Applying a cold compress can soothe inflammation and reduce itching. Over-the-counter hydrocortisone cream may help alleviate symptoms like redness and swelling. If you experience more severe symptoms, such as difficulty breathing or widespread hives, seek medical attention immediately, as these may indicate a severe allergic reaction requiring professional intervention.

Understanding these risks and precautions empowers you to enjoy essential oils safely and confidently. By staying informed and attentive, you can integrate these potent natural remedies into your life with minimal risk, allowing their benefits to enhance your well-being without compromising safety.

## 2.4 PATCH TESTING AND DILUTION RATIOS EXPLAINED

When incorporating essential oils into your routine, understanding how to apply them safely to your skin is vital. A patch test is the first line of defense against unwanted reactions. This simple yet effective step allows you to gauge how your skin will react to a new oil.

To perform a patch test:

1. Start by diluting the essential oil with a suitable carrier oil, such as jojoba or sweet almond oil, known for its gentle properties.
2. Apply a small amount of the diluted oil to a discrete area of your skin, like the inside of your forearm.
3. Cover it with a bandage and leave it undisturbed for 24 hours.
4. After this period, check for any signs of irritation, such as redness or itching. If your skin shows no adverse reaction, proceeding with broader use is likely safe.

Though seemingly simple, this method provides peace of mind and helps prevent discomfort.

The dilution process is critical to ensuring the safe use of essential oils on the skin. Essential oils are highly concentrated and diluting them with a carrier oil reduces the risk of skin irritation. A standard dilution ratio for adults is typically 2-3%, which equals about 12–18 drops of essential oil per ounce of carrier oil. A milder dilution of 1% or even 0.5% is recommended for children or those with sensitive skin, equating to about six drops of essential oil per ounce of carrier oil. These guidelines help ensure the oils remain effective while minimizing potential adverse reactions. Carrier oils dilute crucial oils and add their beneficial properties, enhancing the overall experience.

Several factors can influence the appropriate dilution ratio for you. Skin type plays a significant role; those with sensitive skin may require a higher degree of dilution to avoid irritation. The potency of the essential oil also matters. Some oils, like peppermint or clove, are naturally more intense and should be diluted more than milder oils, like lavender. It's also important to consider the area of application. Delicate regions like the face often require more cautious dilution than less sensitive body areas. Seasonal changes can also affect skin sensitivity, so adjusting your dilution ratio to weather conditions can optimize your experience.

To illustrate:

1. Consider a scenario where you want to create a soothing massage oil.
2. Begin with sweet almond oil as your base, as it nourishes and absorbs well into the skin.
3. For a relaxing blend, add 12 drops of lavender essential oil to one ounce of the carrier oil, achieving a 2% dilution. If making a facial serum, however, you'd opt for a lighter carrier oil like jojoba and use

only six drops of essential oil per ounce to maintain a gentle touch.

These practical examples demonstrate how understanding dilution can enhance your enjoyment and safety when using essential oils. As we conclude this chapter on essential oil safety, the importance of careful application and knowledge becomes apparent. You can confidently integrate essential oils into your daily routine by mastering patch testing and proper dilution. This foundation of safety allows you to explore their numerous benefits without worry. As we move forward, these principles will guide our exploration into essential oils' practical uses and healing properties, paving the way for a deeper understanding and appreciation of their potential in everyday life.

# 3

# ESSENTIAL OILS FOR STRESS RELIEF

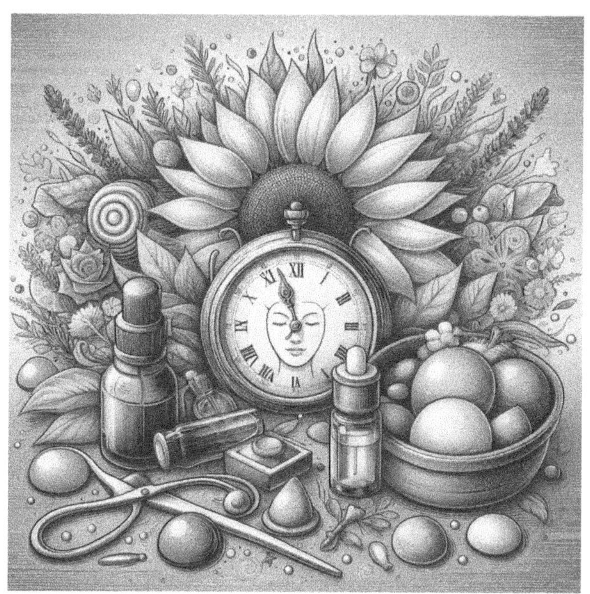

After a demanding day, as you find yourself overwhelmed with uncompleted tasks and pressing deadlines, stress seems to envelop you like a persistent shadow. In these moments, you seek a sliver of solace, an escape from the tight grip of tension. This is the juncture where the remarkable benefits of essential oils come into play, offering a serene retreat from the turmoil. Among the vast array of choices, a select few are particularly renowned for their soothing virtues, each possessing a distinct capability to calm the mind. Lavender, chamomile, and bergamot stand as beacons of tranquility, each imparting its unique essence to aid in your pursuit of peace.

## 3.1 STRESS RELIEF ENHANCEMENT

Lavender oil is the quintessential choice for easing anxiety. Its soft, floral aroma can envelop you in a serene embrace, much like a gentle lullaby. The science behind this calming effect is fascinating. Lavender interacts with the limbic system, the part of your brain that governs emotions and memories. By affecting this area, lavender can reduce stress and promote relaxation. A systematic review and meta-analysis of 21 studies found that lavender significantly lowers stress levels, particularly in the L. angustifolia species (Source 1). This evidence supports its widespread use in stress management programs, especially for those in high-pressure environments like students. Chamomile oil, with its warm, apple-like scent, works similarly, soothing frazzled nerves and encouraging a state of calm. Known for its gentle touch, chamomile has been used for centuries to ease tension and promote rest.

Bergamot oil offers a different relief that uplifts and brightens the mood. Its citrusy aroma is like a ray of sunshine on a cloudy day, dispelling gloom and invigorating the senses. Bergamot's interaction with the limbic system helps to alleviate stress while fostering a sense of joy and positivity. Studies have shown that bergamot can effectively reduce feelings of anxiety and depression, making it a valuable tool for emotional well-being (Source 3). The unique combination of citrus and floral notes in bergamot creates a refreshing scent that can lift your spirits and clear your mind, offering a mental reset.

Incorporating these oils into your routine can be straightforward and rewarding. Direct inhalation is a powerful technique for immediate relief. Inhale deeply from a bottle or use a few drops on a tissue or cotton ball. The aroma will quickly reach your brain, triggering a calming response. Another effective method is topical application, where you dilute the oil with a carrier oil and apply it to pulse points like the wrists, temples, or the back of your neck. This allows the scent to linger and provides a soothing, tactile experience. Additionally, using these oils in a diffuser can create a tranquil atmosphere, filling your space with calming aromas that gently ease your mind.

**Try This: Stress-Relief Inhalation Exercise**

Find a comfortable seat and take a slow, deep breath. Hold a bottle of lavender oil a few inches from your nose. Inhale deeply and exhale slowly. Visualize the tension melting away with each breath. Repeat three times, allowing the calming aroma to envelop you.

These application methods are simple yet effective, offering flexibility in incorporating essential oils into your life. Whether you need a quick mental reset or a more immersive experience, these oils can meet your needs. By understanding how each oil interacts with your body and mind, you can tailor your approach to find the most effective stress relief. With lavender, chamomile, and bergamot by your side, you have natural tools to navigate life's stresses, bringing peace and balance to your everyday moments.

## 3.2 CREATING A RELAXING HOME ATMOSPHERE

The environment you create at home can significantly influence your stress levels. A cluttered space can lead to a cluttered mind, making it difficult to unwind. Your home should be a sanctuary where you can leave the day's troubles at the door. One of the most potent elements in setting this atmosphere is scent. The right aroma can evoke calm and serenity, helping you relax and recharge. Essential oils offer a natural way to infuse your space with soothing scents. Their impact on mood regulation is profound, as scent is intricately linked to our emotions and memories.

Using essential oils in a diffuser is an effective way to disperse calming aromas throughout your home. Consider a blend of lavender, sandalwood, and ylang-ylang for evening relaxation. This combination promotes a peaceful environment, encouraging relaxation and restful sleep. Lavender brings its gentle floral notes, which are known for reducing tension. Sandalwood adds a grounding, woody aroma that calms the mind, while ylang-ylang introduces a sweet, exotic scent that lifts the spirit. Together, these oils create a harmonious blend that transforms your home into a haven of tranquility.

Integrating essential oils into your daily routine can provide continuous stress relief. Start your day with eucalyptus oil in the shower. Its refreshing aroma clears the mind and energizes the body, preparing you for the day ahead. Add a few drops to your shower floor and let the steam carry the scent. As the day winds down, incorporate calming oils into your bedtime routine. Diffuse a relaxing blend in your bedroom or add drops to your pillow. This practice signals your body that it's time to unwind and fosters a sense of continuity, creating a soothing ritual you can look forward to each night.

Besides scent, other sensory elements like lighting and music are crucial in enhancing relaxation. Soft lighting creates a cozy ambiance, signaling your brain to relax. Use dimmable lights or lamps with warm bulbs to set a gentle evening glow. Pairing this with essential oils can amplify the calming effect, making your space feel even more inviting. Music is another powerful tool. Craft playlists filled with soothing melodies or nature sounds to accompany your aromatherapy session. The combination of pleasant scents and peaceful sounds can help drown out the noise of the day, allowing you to sink into a state of deep relaxation.

**Try This: Evening Relaxation Routine**

Allocate 20 minutes before bedtime for relaxation. Disconnect by placing your digital devices in a different room. Dim the lights to foster a tranquil ambiance, then turn on your diffuser, releasing a calming blend of lavender, sandalwood, and ylang-ylang oils into the air. Settle into a cozy spot and allow the gentle melodies of rain or ocean waves to fill the room, enveloping you in a peaceful auditory embrace. With closed eyes, focus on taking deep, measured breaths, immersing yourself in the harmonious dance of fragrance and sound. This routine is a gateway to more profound relaxation and a catalyst for improved sleep quality.

Creating a relaxing home atmosphere is about engaging all your senses. You can craft a space that supports your well-being by thoughtfully combining scent, lighting, and sound. These elements work together to reduce stress and promote peace, making your home a true refuge from the outside world. The small changes you make can profoundly impact your mood and stress levels, allowing you to unwind and rejuvenate fully.

## 3.3 AROMATHERAPY TECHNIQUES FOR STRESS REDUCTION

At its core, aromatherapy taps into the profound connection between scent and the human psyche. It's a practice that uses essential oils to enhance physical and emotional well-being. By engaging the olfactory senses, aromatherapy can influence mood and reduce stress. This method has been used for centuries, rooted in the belief that natural plant extracts hold the power to heal and calm. Imagine your senses awakening to the gentle aroma wafting from a diffuser or the subtle floral notes in a warm bath. These are not mere scents but tools to alleviate stress and foster relaxation.

One of the simplest yet most effective aromatherapy techniques is steam inhalation. This involves adding a few drops of essential oil into a bowl of hot water and then inhaling the steam. The aromatic molecules travel through the nasal passages, reaching the brain swiftly, offering immediate calming effects. This technique is excellent for quick stress relief, as the warmth of the steam coupled with the scent of oils like eucalyptus or peppermint can open airways and clear the mind. Another beloved practice is incorporating essential oils into bath soaks. Combining warm water and soothing scents creates a tranquil environment where stress melts away. Oils like lavender or chamomile in your bath can help relax tense muscles and calm a racing mind, offering a holistic approach to stress reduction.

Aromatherapy seamlessly complements mindfulness practices, amplifying their soothing benefits. When used during meditation, essential oils can deepen concentration and promote a sense of peace. Oils such as frankincense or sandalwood are particularly effective, grounding the mind and allowing you to focus inward. Integrating essential oils into yoga practice is another powerful method. The mindful movements of yoga, combined with the therapeutic scents, can enhance your relaxation. Oils like lemongrass or orange can be diffused in the practice space, invigorating the senses while you stretch and breathe. This harmonious blend of aroma and motion can elevate your practice, making it more enriching and healing.

Real-life stories attest to the transformative power of aromatherapy. Consider the experience of a yoga instructor who began using essential oils in her classes. She noticed a marked difference in her students' engagement and stress levels. Adding diffused lavender during savasana, the final resting pose, helped her students relax more deeply. They reported feeling more centered and less anxious after class, attributing their improved mood to the calming aromas.

These testimonials underscore how essential oils, when used mindfully, can enhance existing stress-reduction practices.

Aromatherapy offers a versatile toolkit for stress relief. The possibilities are endless, whether you choose steam inhalation for quick relief, a luxurious bath soak, or using oils in mindfulness practices. The simplicity and accessibility of these techniques mean they can be easily incorporated into daily life, offering a natural and pleasant way to manage stress. By embracing these methods, you can create a more balanced and harmonious lifestyle, one where the calming influence of essential oils supports you in navigating the challenges of the day.

## 3.4 PERSONALIZED BLENDS FOR EMOTIONAL BALANCE

Imagine the power of crafting a scent that feels like it was made just for you, one that lifts your spirits on a dreary day or grounds you when life feels chaotic. Creating your own essential oil blends offers this kind of personalized support for emotional balance. It begins with understanding your scent preferences and the profiles of various oils. Each oil carries distinct properties and aromas that can evoke specific emotions or states of mind. For instance, citrus oils like lemon or grapefruit are renowned for their ability to uplift and energize. Their bright, zesty notes can bring positivity through the mental fog. Frankincense, on the other hand, offers a sense of grounding and focus. Its deep, resinous aroma can help anchor your thoughts, making it an excellent choice when you need to concentrate or meditate.

To start crafting blends that suit your emotional needs, it's helpful to familiarize yourself with the emotional properties of different oils. Think of them as a palette of scents, each with its emotional signature. Citrus oils can brighten your mood and are invigorating, perfect for those days when you feel sluggish. In contrast, woody oils like cedarwood or vetiver bring a calming, stabilizing effect, ideal for moments when you're overwhelmed and need a sense of peace. Florals, such as rose or jasmine, are often associated with feelings of love and comfort, enveloping you in a sense of warmth and care. By aligning these properties with your scent preferences, you can create a blend that resonates with your current emotional state and desired outcome.

Blending oils is both an art and a science. It involves choosing complementary scents and considering the ratios to achieve a balanced aroma. A typical starting point is the 3:2:1 ratio, which often works well for blending multiple oils. This ratio allows the dominant oil to lead, supported by the secondary and base oils, creating a harmonious blend. For example, crafting a calming blend might use three parts lavender, two parts bergamot, and one part frankincense. This combination provides a soothing aroma with depth and complexity. Using rollerball bottles can make application easy and portable. Fill the bottle halfway with your chosen blend and top with a carrier oil such as fractionated coconut oil. This setup dilutes the essential oils and makes applying the blend to pulse points convenient whenever you need a quick emotional reset.

Experimentation is a key part of finding your perfect blend. Each person's response to scents is unique and shaped by personal experiences and associations. Keeping an aromatherapy journal can be a valuable tool in this process. Documenting your blends and their effects helps you refine your creations—note which oils you used, the ratios, and how the blend made you feel. Over time, you may notice patterns or preferences emerging, guiding you in fine-tuning your blends for maximum impact. Reflecting on your emotional state before and after using a blend can also provide insights into its effectiveness. This practice enhances your blending skills and deepens your understanding of how scents influence your mood and emotions.

As you navigate the world of personalized blends, remember that there's no right or wrong way to create your unique scent. It's about exploring what feels suitable for you and what brings balance to your emotional landscape. With each experiment, you're not just creating a scent; you're crafting a tool that supports your well-being, tailored to your needs. The beauty of this process lies in its flexibility and personal nature, allowing you to adapt and adjust as you grow and change. Embrace the journey of discovery and enjoy the empowerment of creating a blend that feels like your own personal sanctuary. Your blends are an extension of yourself, a fragrant reflection of your inner world and the balance you seek.

Personalizing your essential oil blends opens a world of customization, allowing you to tailor solutions to your emotional needs. As you explore these blends, consider how they can fit into your broader self-care practices. With a deeper understanding of your emotional landscape, you can curate blends that enhance your daily life. This chapter has laid the groundwork for using essential oils to manage stress and foster emotional balance. We will explore how these oils can improve sleep quality as we move forward, offering a natural way to unwind and recharge.

# 4

# ENHANCING SLEEP QUALITY

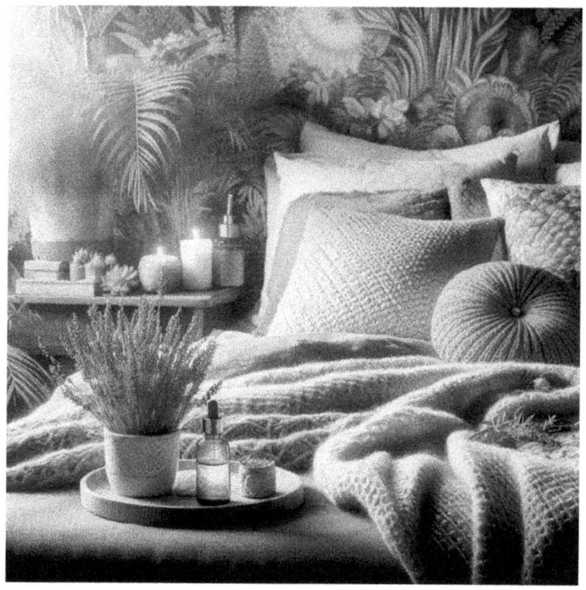

Imagine unwinding in the tranquility of the evening after a day filled with activity and stress. The desire for sleep is strong, but it seems just out of reach. This scenario is all too familiar for many adults, who are awake with thoughts racing. Essential oils emerge as a gentle, natural solution to this widespread issue, leading you toward the peaceful sleep you long for. Their calming aromas have the power to transform your bedroom into a sanctuary of rest, priming your mind and body for a night of deep, rejuvenating sleep.

## 4.1 BEDTIME ROUTINE

Establishing a consistent bedtime routine is a cornerstone of good sleep hygiene. Just as children thrive on routine, adults also benefit from a structured approach to winding down. By setting a specific bedtime and wake-up time, your body learns to anticipate sleep, aligning your internal clock with your lifestyle. This regularity signals your body to prepare for rest, making it easier to fall asleep and wake up refreshed. Consider this routine a signal to your brain that it's time to let go of the day's stresses and embrace relaxation.

Incorporating essential oils into your evening rituals can significantly enhance this process. Lavender oil, with its calming properties, is a beautiful choice. Diffuse it in your bedroom about an hour before you plan to sleep. The gentle aroma fills the room, creating a tranquil atmosphere that encourages relaxation. This practice soothes your senses and helps establish a clear association between the scent of lavender and sleep, reinforcing your body's natural sleep cues. Similarly, adding a few drops of chamomile oil to a warm bath can be a luxurious way to unwind. The warm water relaxes tense muscles, while the chamomile gently calms the mind, setting the stage for a peaceful slumber.

The power of olfactory cues in relaxation cannot be overstated. Our sense of smell is directly linked to the limbic system, the part of the brain that governs emotions and memories. Certain scents can evoke feelings of calm and safety, making them powerful tools in preparing the mind for sleep. Essential oils tap into this connection, providing a natural way to influence your emotional state. By consciously engaging these olfactory cues, you create an environment conducive to relaxation, allowing your mind to transition smoothly from the busyness of the day to the tranquility of night.

Personalizing your bedtime routine is key to ensuring it fits seamlessly into your life. Everyone's preferences and schedules are different, so it's essential to tailor your rituals to what feels most comforting and effective for you. Journaling with calming scents can be a grounding practice. Light a candle infused with your favorite essential oil and let its aroma accompany you as you reflect on your day. This practice helps process thoughts and creates a calming pre-sleep ritual. Listening to soothing music while diffusing essential oils can also be a delightful addition to your routine. Choose melodies that relax you and pair them with oils like sandalwood or cedarwood for a deeply calming experience.

**Reflection Activity: Designing Your Sleep Sanctuary**

Pause and envision your perfect sanctuary for sleep. Which aromas, melodies, and textures summon tranquility for you? Integrate these soothing elements into your nightly routine to cultivate a serene atmosphere. Reflect on specific adjustments you can make to transform your bedroom into a haven of relaxation and enhanced sleep quality. Suggestions include organizing and purifying your space to reduce clutter, which can disturb the mind. Consider the arrangement of furniture for optimal flow and comfort, the selection of bedding that invites touch with its softness, and the removal of distractions from your nightstand and dresser. Envision a minimalist, peaceful environment that supports your journey to restful sleep.

You create a series of habits and a sanctuary for sleep by thoughtfully designing your bedtime routine. This space becomes a refuge where you can retreat from the day's demands and focus on rest and renewal. As you experiment with different oils and practices, you'll discover what works best for you, gradually building a routine uniquely suited to your needs. This personal touch transforms your sleep routine into an intentional self-care practice that nurtures both body and mind as you drift into restorative sleep.

## 4.2 BEST OILS FOR RESTORATIVE SLEEP

Certain essential oils stand out for their remarkable properties when achieving a restful night's sleep. Among these, vetiver oil is often highlighted for its ability to promote deep relaxation. It is known for its earthy and grounding aroma; vetiver works by calming the nervous system, making it an ideal choice for those nights when your mind refuses to quiet down. The science behind vetiver's effects lies in its interaction with neurotransmitters that influence relaxation. Its compounds can help reduce anxiety and stress, creating a tranquil state conducive to sleep. To make the most of vetiver, apply it to the pulse points on your wrists or the back of your neck before bed. Dilute it with a carrier oil to prevent irritation and enjoy its calming benefits. For those who prefer wearable aromatherapy, using a diffuser bracelet infused with vetiver oil can provide continuous exposure to its soothing scent throughout the night.

Cedarwood oil is another excellent option for sleep support, particularly appreciated for its grounding and stabilizing properties. Its warm, woody aroma is not just pleasant; it's also profoundly comforting. Cedarwood oil interacts with the brain's limbic system, which regulates emotions and memory. This interaction can help quiet racing thoughts and ease emotional tension, creating an environment ripe for restful sleep. Cedarwood's sedative effects are thought to be due to its high concentration of sesquiterpenes, compounds that help promote relaxation and decrease overactivity in the brain. For optimal use, apply cedarwood oil to your temples and pulse points. Its grounding aroma can also be effectively used in a diffuser necklace, allowing you to carry the calming scent as you prepare for bedtime.

Selecting the right essential oil for sleep involves considering your specific challenges and preferences. If you struggle with an overactive mind, vetiver might be your go-to. Its ability to soothe and calm makes it perfect for those who find it difficult to switch off after a long day. On the other hand, if your sleep troubles stem from emotional unrest or anxiety, cedarwood can provide the emotional grounding you need to feel secure and relaxed. Experiment with both oils to see which resonates most with you. Some people even find that combining them enhances their effects, creating a personalized blend that addresses physical and emotional sleep barriers. Remember to patch-test new oils to ensure they don't irritate your skin, especially when trying them in new applications.

Incorporating these oils into your nightly routine can transform your sleep experience. The subtle yet powerful aromas can create an oasis of calm, helping you transition smoothly from the bustle of the day to the serenity of night. Making essential oils a part of your bedtime ritual enhances your sleep quality and invests in your overall well-being. By choosing vetiver, cedarwood, or a combination of both, these essential oils offer a natural way to achieve the deep, rejuvenating sleep your body craves.

## 4.3 BLENDING OILS FOR SLEEP-INDUCING EFFECTS

Creating your essential oil blends can be a deeply rewarding process, especially when crafting those aimed at enhancing sleep. The key lies in understanding how different oils complement each other, forming a harmonious blend that maximizes their benefits. Balancing top, middle, and base notes is at the heart of this process. Top notes are those first fleeting impressions, often bright and uplifting, like the refreshing scent of bergamot. Middle notes, such as lavender, provide a grounding presence, forming the heart of the blend with a soothing, lasting aroma. Base notes, like frankincense, add depth and longevity, anchoring the scent while providing a calming foundation.

When combined effectively, oils can create a positive effect, where the blend is more potent than the sum of its parts. For instance, pairing lavender, bergamot, and frankincense creates a comprehensive sleep aid. Lavender's calming properties are well-documented, providing a sense of peace. With its citrusy brightness, bergamot helps alleviate anxiety and lift the mood, making it easier to let go of the day's worries. Frankincense, known for its grounding and introspective qualities, helps deepen the relaxation experience. Together, these oils form a blend that smells divine and works powerfully to prepare the body and mind for restful sleep.

For those looking to try their hand at blending, here's a recipe to get started: The "Sweet Dreams" blend. This blend combines lavender, marjoram, and sandalwood. Lavender, as always, brings its calming floral scent. Marjoram adds a warm, herby note that soothes nerves and promotes emotional balance. Sandalwood, with its rich, woody aroma, provides a grounding effect, perfect for quieting a restless mind. To create this blend, start with three drops of lavender, two drops of marjoram, and one drop of sandalwood, adjusting the ratios to suit your personal preference. This blend can be diffused in the bedroom or added to a carrier oil for a relaxing bedtime massage.

Experimentation is encouraged in the art of blending. Each person's sense of smell and emotional responses to scents are unique, making it essential to find what works best for you. Keep a journal to note which blends are most effective, recording the specific oils and ratios used and your observations on their impact. Over time, you may notice patterns in which oils or combinations offer the most significant benefit. Adjusting the ratios based on scent preference or the desired effect can lead to a genuinely personalized blend. Perhaps you prefer a stronger presence of lavender, or maybe you find sandalwood's grounding aroma particularly comforting. These adjustments allow you to tailor blends to your specific sleep needs and personal tastes.

Creating these blends is both a science and an art, balancing precision with creativity. As you explore, remember that there is no one-size-fits-all solution. The beauty lies in discovering what resonates with you, offering tranquility and support as you seek a peaceful night's sleep. Each blend reflects your journey toward relaxation, capturing the essence of your unique path to well-being.

## 4.4 DIY PILLOW SPRAYS AND SLEEP MASKS

Creating your sleep aids with essential oils can be both therapeutic and empowering. When you make personalized sleep products, you tailor them to your preferences, ensuring they meet your specific needs. DIY pillow sprays, for instance, allow you to craft a blend that resonates with your senses, setting the stage for a restful night. These sprays are not just about fragrance; they are about creating an inviting sleep environment that soothes and calms.

To begin, gather your materials: a small spray bottle, distilled water, and witch hazel. Distilled water serves as the base, ensuring the purity of your spray. Witch hazel acts as a natural preservative, extending the life of your creation while adding a subtle, refreshing scent. Mix in your selected essential oils next. While lavender and chamomile stand out for their soothing effects, don't hesitate to experiment with alternatives such as sandalwood or marjoram to create a distinctive mixture. Start by filling your spray bottle halfway with distilled water. Add a tablespoon of witch hazel to stabilize the mixture. Then, introduce 10-15 drops of essential oil, adjusting the quantity based on your preference for a stronger or milder scent. Shake well to blend the ingredients.

This custom pillow spray can mist your pillows, bed linens, or even pajamas before sleep, enveloping you in a cloud of tranquility. The gentle mist carries the oils' soothing aromas, engaging your senses and signaling to your body that it's time to relax. Incorporating this simple ritual into your nightly routine creates a consistent cue for your mind to unwind.

Sleep masks infused with essential oils offer another layer of relaxation. These masks combine the benefits of darkness and scent, enhancing your ability to fall asleep quickly and deeply. By blocking out light, the mask encourages your body to produce melatonin, a hormone that regulates sleep. When infused with calming oils like chamomile or lavender, the mask provides an added sensory experience. To infuse a mask:

1. Apply a few drops of essential oil onto a cotton pad or a small piece of fabric.
2. Allow it to dry slightly to prevent any direct contact with your skin.
3. Place this inside a pocket within the mask or attach it to the outer fabric. As you wear the mask, your body's warmth will gently release the oils' aroma, creating a cocoon of calm.

If you're experiencing outside noise, consider using soft earplugs or listening to white noise for a more peaceful environment. Encouraging creativity in these DIY projects can transform them into a personal exploration of scent and relaxation. Experiment with different oils to find combinations that resonate with you. Your favorite calming oils might include ylang-ylang for its floral sweetness or cedarwood for its earthy grounding. Don't hesitate to incorporate dried herbs like lavender buds or chamomile flowers, which can enhance your creations' scent and aesthetics. Placing these herbs inside a sachet or a mask can provide a subtle, continuous fragrance.

This experimentation is about discovering what works best for your sleep needs and preferences. Everyone's sleep environment is unique, and these DIY projects allow you to tailor yours to be as relaxing as possible. Creating these aids can be meditative and rewarding, offering a deeper connection to the sleep process. You build a nurturing and effective routine by engaging with the materials and scents.

The chapter concludes with an invitation to explore these DIY sleep aids further. By crafting your own pillow sprays and sleep masks, you can enhance your sleep quality and personalize your environment. As you continue reading, consider how these practices might integrate with the broader themes of natural wellness explored in the next chapter.

5

# ESSENTIAL OILS FOR MUSCLE RECOVERY

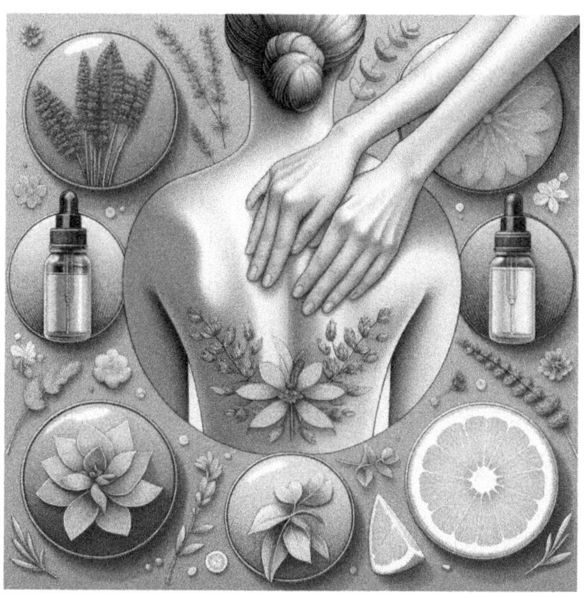

Visualize the profound relief and satisfaction of completing a rigorous workout: your muscles are tired but gratifying, signaling a job well done. Now, the prospect of recovery looms near, courtesy of nature's healing treasures. Essential oils, renowned for their soothing and therapeutic properties, stand ready to provide effective post-exercise care. These potent natural extracts work wonders in easing muscle tension, diminishing inflammation, and speeding up recovery. This helps you return to your activities with greater strength and resilience and enriches your self-care regimen with a holistic touch. As you delve into the myriad benefits of essential oils for muscle recovery, embrace them as a vital component of your wellness arsenal, offering a natural and nurturing path to enhance your physical health.

## 5.1 POST-WORKOUT RECOVERY OILS

Among the essential oils known for their ability to support muscle recovery, peppermint oil stands out due to its cooling and tension-reducing properties. Peppermint oil contains menthol, a compound known for its analgesic and anti-inflammatory effects. When applied to sore muscles, menthol creates a cooling sensation that can help alleviate pain and reduce swelling. This makes peppermint oil particularly useful when your muscles feel overworked or strained. It's refreshing aroma also provides a mental boost, invigorating your senses and helping to clear any workout fog. To use peppermint oil effectively, consider applying it directly to the affected area using a rollerball applicator. This method allows for precise application and ensures that the oil is absorbed quickly, providing targeted relief where you need it most.

Eucalyptus oil is another powerful ally in muscle recovery, prized for its ability to alleviate muscle aches and inflammation. This oil contains eucalyptol, a compound with anti-inflammatory properties that can help soothe irritated muscles. The cooling effect of eucalyptus oil, like that of peppermint, can provide relief from muscle pain, making it an ideal choice for post-workout care. Eucalyptus oil is particularly beneficial for those engaging in activities that place significant muscle stress, such as weightlifting or endurance sports. For a more immersive experience, consider adding a few drops of eucalyptus oil to a warm compress. Apply the compress to the sore area, allowing the heat to work with the oil, relaxing the muscles and promoting healing.

Athletes and trainers often rely on these oils to enhance their recovery routines. Consider the testimony of a marathon runner who incorporates peppermint oil into her post-race rituals. After a long-distance run, her muscles feel fatigued and sore, but applying peppermint oil gives immediate relief. The cooling sensation helps to reduce inflammation, allowing her to recover faster and prepare for her next training session. Similarly, a personal trainer shares how eucalyptus oil has become a staple in his kit. He recommends it to clients who experience muscle soreness after intense weightlifting sessions. The oil helps reduce pain and aids in preventing further injury by encouraging relaxation and flexibility in the muscles.

**Reflection Section: Crafting Your Recovery Routine**

Take a moment to think about your current post-exercise routine. Consider how incorporating essential oils might enhance your recovery experience. Jot down a few ideas on integrating peppermint or eucalyptus oil into your regimen. Whether through a quick rollerball application or a soothing compress, these oils can help you recover more effectively.

By integrating essential oils like peppermint and eucalyptus into your recovery routine, you support your muscles and engage in a holistic approach to fitness. These oils work with your body's natural processes, promoting healing and reducing discomfort. As you continue to explore the benefits of essential oils, you'll find that they offer a versatile and effective solution for maintaining your active lifestyle.

## 5.2 BLENDING FOR INFLAMMATION AND SORENESS

The art of blending essential oils to combat inflammation and soreness is science and intuition. By understanding how different oils interact, you can create powerful combinations that enhance the individual properties of each oil. Start by considering the combination of wintergreen and frankincense. Wintergreen, with its high concentration of methyl salicylate, offers potent anti-inflammatory properties, making it ideal for reducing swelling and easing joint pain. Frankincense complements this by promoting relaxation and reducing stress, which can often exacerbate physical discomfort. Together, these oils create a blend that targets inflammation and calms the mind, assisting in a holistic recovery process.

Blending oils is much like crafting a fine dish—the ingredients must complement each other. Black pepper and ginger are another dynamic duo, offering a warming effect that can soothe sore muscles. Black pepper oil is known for its ability to enhance circulation, which helps to flush out toxins and bring fresh oxygen to tired muscles. Conversely, ginger adds a warming sensation that penetrates deeply, relieving stiffness and tension. Combining black pepper and ginger can be especially advantageous following a strenuous workout or when managing chronic muscle pain, offering immediate relief and long-term benefits.

Creating your blend for muscle relief allows you to tailor the experience to your specific needs. Consider the "Soothe and Heal" blend, which combines lavender, marjoram, and rosemary oils. Lavender offers a calming effect, easing both physical and mental tension. Marjoram is renowned for its ability to relax muscle spasms, making it perfect for soothing sore muscles. Rosemary adds a refreshing touch, enhancing circulation and reducing pain. To prepare this blend, mix five drops of lavender, four drops of marjoram, and three drops of rosemary in a small glass bottle. Add a carrier oil such as jojoba to dilute the blend, ensuring it's gentle on the skin while still potent enough to offer relief.

Customization is key when it comes to essential oil blends. You can adjust the ratios based on your preferences and specific recovery needs. If you find minty oils like peppermint cooling sensation too intense, you can balance it with warming oils like ginger or clove. This flexibility allows you to create a blend that feels right for you. Additionally, consider the benefits of different carrier oils. Jojoba oil is excellent for sensitive skin, as it closely mimics the body's natural oils. Sweet almond oil, rich in vitamins and nutrients, adds a nourishing element that can enhance the overall experience.

**Interactive Element: Create Your Custom Muscle Relief Blend**

Take a moment to think about the types of muscle soreness you experience most frequently. Do you prefer a cooling or warming sensation? Use this information to guide your blend creation. Mix and match oils in small quantities until you find a combination that's just right. Record the recipes you create and note how each blend affects your soreness and recovery.

These personalized blends offer a unique way to support your body's recovery and well-being. By experimenting with different combinations, you can discover what works best for you, crafting effective and enjoyable solutions. The creative and therapeutic process invites you to explore and learn while caring for your body.

## 5.3 MASSAGE TECHNIQUES WITH ESSENTIAL OILS

Incorporating massage into your recovery routine is a powerful way to promote muscle healing and relaxation. When combined with essential oils, massage becomes even more effective, as the oils enhance the therapeutic experience by soothing tired muscles and reducing tension. The physical act of massage increases blood circulation, which aids in delivering nutrients and oxygen to tissues, accelerating the healing process. This improved circulation helps flush out metabolic waste products accumulated during exercise, reducing soreness and stiffness. By integrating essential oils into massage, their distinct properties amplify the recovery process, offering anti-inflammatory and pain-relieving advantages. This combination enhances the holistic nature of massage as a full-spectrum strategy for muscle wellness.

To perform an effective muscle recovery massage, start with circular motions, ideal for relaxing deep tissue. These movements focus on applying pressure to specific areas, working out knots, and improving flexibility. Begin with gentle pressure and gradually increase as the muscles warm up, allowing the oils to penetrate deeply. Following circular motions, incorporate long strokes, which aid in lymphatic drainage. These strokes are designed to encourage the movement of lymph fluid throughout the body, helping to remove toxins and reduce swelling. Use these strokes upward towards the heart, applying more pressure on the upstroke and lighter on the return. This technique enhances relaxation and contributes to detoxification, fostering a sense of well-being.

The choice of carrier oil is crucial in massage, as it dilutes essential oils, ensuring safety and effectiveness. Sweet almond oil is popular due to its light texture and rich nutrient profile, making it easily absorbed by the skin without leaving a greasy residue. It's packed with vitamins A and E, which nourish and hydrate the skin while providing a smooth glide during massage. Grapeseed oil is another excellent option, known for its light texture and high linoleic acid content, which is beneficial for repairing and rejuvenating skin. Both oils enhance the overall experience, allowing essential oils to be applied safely while delivering therapeutic benefits. Mixing a few drops of your chosen essential oil with a tablespoon of carrier oil creates a balanced blend that can be massaged into the skin, ensuring optimal absorption and effectiveness.

Expert massage therapists often emphasize the importance of targeting specific muscle groups to maximize recovery. For instance, when addressing soreness in larger muscle groups like the quadriceps or hamstrings, focus on broad, sweeping strokes covering the entire muscle. This approach ensures even pressure distribution and allows the oils to work effectively across a wider area. Use your fingertips to apply gentle, circular pressure for smaller, more intricate areas like the neck or shoulders. This technique helps release tension and knots that can accumulate in these regions, often exacerbated by stress or poor posture. Additionally, incorporating stretching into your massage routine can further enhance recovery. Gently stretching muscles after massage helps maintain flexibility and prevent stiffness, promoting long-term muscle health.

To optimize your massage experience, consider setting the scene with dim lighting and calming music, creating a relaxing atmosphere. This holistic approach addresses physical discomfort and fosters mental tranquility, allowing you to unwind and fully reap the benefits of massage and aromatherapy. Integrating these techniques into your routine can enhance muscle recovery, improve flexibility, and support overall well-being.

## 5.4 CREATING MUSCLE-SOOTHING BATH BLENDS

Imagine sinking into a warm bath after a strenuous day, feeling the tension in your muscles dissolve. Bath therapy, with the addition of essential oils, offers a holistic way to soothe sore muscles and promote relaxation. The combination of heat and aromatic oils creates an environment where your body can release stress and restore balance. The warm water opens your pores, allowing the oils to penetrate deeply and work their magic. This soothing ritual is not just about physical relief; it provides a mental escape, giving you peace and tranquility.

Creating a muscle-relaxing bath blend is simple and rewarding. One effective recipe is the "Relax and Renew" bath soak, which combines Epsom salts, lavender, and juniper berry oils. Start by drawing a warm bath and adding one cup of Epsom salt. Epsom salts are rich in magnesium, a mineral that plays a crucial role in muscle function. Magnesium helps to reduce muscle stiffness and inflammation, making it an ideal companion for recovery. Next, add five drops of lavender oil for its calming and pain-relieving properties. Lavender eases muscle tension and helps calm the mind, enhancing the overall relaxation experience. Finally, include three drops of juniper berry oil. Known for its detoxifying effects, juniper berry helps flush out toxins that accumulate in the muscles after exercise, further aiding recovery.

The choice to incorporate Epsom salts is not just about tradition; it's rooted in science. Magnesium, found abundantly in Epsom salts, is essential for muscle relaxation and recovery. It helps regulate muscle contractions and reduces lactic acid buildup, which can cause soreness. Soaking in a bath enriched with Epsom salts lets your body absorb magnesium through the skin, directly targeting muscle stiffness and discomfort. This method is both efficient and gentle, offering relief without the need for additional supplements or medications. The salts also have a natural exfoliating effect, leaving your skin feeling soft and rejuvenated.

Personalizing your bath ritual can transform it into a profoundly enriching experience. Consider setting the scene with soothing music and dim lighting to enhance the atmosphere. Choose a playlist with gentle melodies or nature sounds that relax you, and let it play softly in the background. Lighting a few candles can add a warm, calming glow, turning your bathroom into a sanctuary of relaxation. As you sink into the tub, take a moment to breathe deeply, inhaling the aromatic steam that rises from the water. This simple act of mindfulness can help center your thoughts, allowing you to fully embrace your bath's restorative power.

Another way to personalize your bath is by experimenting with different essential oils to find the best combination. You may prefer the refreshing scent of eucalyptus or the comforting warmth of ginger. Each oil brings unique benefits, inviting you to tailor your bath to match your mood or specific recovery goals. Mixing your favorite oils can create a signature blend that resonates with you, turning each bath into a ritual of self-care and rejuvenation. The process of trial and error while discovering what works best for you can be both fun and enlightening.

As you cultivate this bath ritual, remember that it's not just about physical recovery; it's an opportunity to nurture your mind and spirit. By taking the time to care for yourself in this way, you acknowledge the importance of balance and well-being. This holistic approach to recovery supports your muscles and overall health, creating a foundation upon which you can build a lifestyle of wellness and vitality.

Embrace the simplicity of this practice, and let it become a cherished part of your routine.

In exploring the soothing potential of bath blends, you tap into a timeless tradition of healing and relaxation. With their natural properties, essential oils enhance this experience, offering a path to recovery that feels both luxurious and accessible. As you continue on this journey of discovery, you'll find that the benefits of essential oils extend far beyond muscle recovery, touching every aspect of your well-being. The next chapter will explore how these oils can support respiratory health, offering relief and comfort in every breath.

# 6

# BREATHING EASIER WITH ESSENTIAL OILS

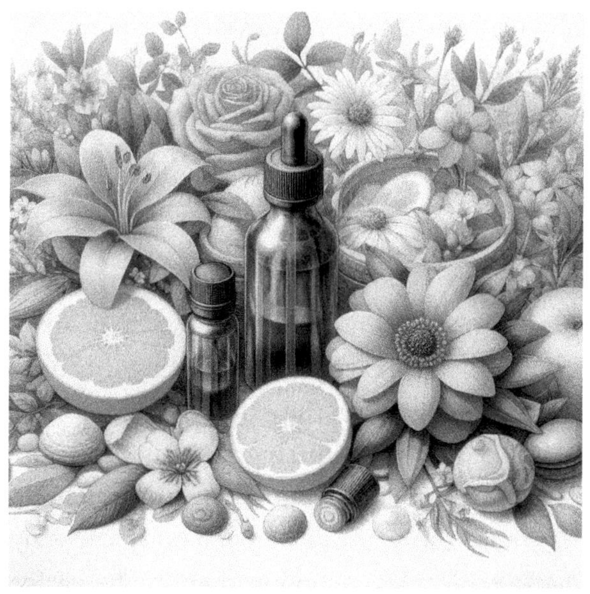

Waking up to the sensation of a stuffy nose and struggling for a comfortable breath is a distressing start to anyone's day. This discomfort, a familiar foe during the chill of winter or the bloom of spring, demands swift and effective relief. Within these moments, the power of essential oils shines; these concentrated plant essences offer a natural, potent solution to the woes of respiratory congestion. By leveraging their unique properties, essential oils act as invaluable allies in the quest for respiratory wellness. They provide the much-needed clarity of breath and comfort, transforming your day from discomfort to ease and relief.

## 6.1 ESSENTIAL OILS FOR RESPIRATORY HEALTH

Embarking on the journey of creating your essential oil blend can be both empowering and therapeutic. To begin, consider starting with a base of eucalyptus and peppermint oils, renowned for their respiratory benefits. A recommended initial ratio is ten drops of eucalyptus oil to 5 drops of peppermint oil. These quantities provide a balanced starting point, delivering the sharp clarity of eucalyptus and peppermint's cooling relief. Select a carrier oil that aligns with your preferences and skin type. Popular choices include almond, coconut, or jojoba oil, known for their gentle and nourishing properties. Integrate the essential oils into one ounce of your chosen carrier oil, ensuring a thorough mix. This diluted blend ensures the potent essential oils are safe for skin application, maximizing benefits and minimizing irritation risk. This blend is most effective when applied to the chest, where the warmth of your body can help diffuse the aromatic molecules, allowing them to be easily inhaled and providing direct respiratory support. Applying before bedtime or at the first sign of congestion can help manage symptoms and promote better sleep. It's also beneficial during the day, especially in environments that may trigger respiratory discomfort. Maintaining a usage journal can be invaluable to tailor this blend to your needs. Record the effects of the blend on your respiratory symptoms, noting any changes in congestion, ease of breathing, or overall comfort. Adjust the ratio of eucalyptus to peppermint based on your observations. Some may find greater relief with a higher concentration of peppermint, while others might prefer the dominant freshness of eucalyptus. This iterative process allows you to refine your blend over time, creating a uniquely effective, personalized remedy for you. Integrating eucalyptus and peppermint oils into your wellness routine offers a proactive approach to managing respiratory health. With their combined properties, these oils work synergistically to clear airways, reduce congestion, and soothe irritation, facilitating breathing and enhancing overall comfort. This natural solution supports your body's respiratory functions, empowering you to breathe more easily and enjoy a higher quality of life.

## 6.2 DIY DIFFUSER BLENDS FOR SINUS RELIEF

Imagine entering a room where the air feels fresh and clear, each breath easier than the last. This is the promise of using a diffuser with essential oils, a simple tool that can make a big difference in how we breathe. Diffusers work by dispersing essential oils into the air, allowing you to benefit from their properties continuously. This continuous release of therapeutic compounds can help alleviate sinus congestion and promote clear breathing, significantly impacting your comfort, especially during allergy season or when battling a cold. By filling the air with these natural aromas, diffusers create an environment that supports respiratory health, offering relief right where you need it.

Creating your diffuser blends tailored to sinus relief is practical and rewarding. A popular blend, known as the "Breathe Easy" blend, combines eucalyptus, rosemary, and lemon essential oils. With its fresh, camphoraceous scent, eucalyptus pairs well with rosemary's herbal notes, known for its decongestant and clearing effects. Lemon adds a bright, uplifting aroma, which can help boost your mood while you clear your airways. To make this blend, add three drops of eucalyptus oil, two drops of rosemary oil, and one drop of lemon oil to your diffuser. This combination works together to open nasal passages and ease breathing, offering both physical and emotional comfort.

Consider the best practices for their use to get the most out of your diffuser blends. The optimal diffusion time is typically 15 to 30 minutes per hour. This allows the oils to effectively permeate the air without overwhelming your senses. Setting your diffuser to intermittent mode helps maintain a consistent level of aroma, giving you sustained relief over time. Positioning the diffuser is key to maximizing its benefits. Place it in a central location within the room, ideally at a height where the mist can disperse evenly. If you're using it in a bedroom, placing the diffuser on a nightstand can help you benefit from the soothing aromas as you rest.

Experimentation with diffuser blends is encouraged, as it allows you to tailor the experience to suit your personal preferences and needs. Adjust the strength of the scent by varying the number of drops you use. If you prefer a more subtle aroma, reduce the number of drops or add more if you like a more substantial presence. Incorporating your favorite oils can also enhance your blend. Adding a drop of lavender for its calming effects or peppermint for its crisp, refreshing scent might suit you better. The beauty of creating your blends is its freedom, allowing you to find the perfect combination that resonates with you.

**Interactive Element: Create Your Own Sinus Relief Blend**

Take a moment to jot down a few of your favorite essential oils. Consider their scents and how they make you feel. Experiment by mixing small amounts in a bowl, noting which combinations you enjoy most. Record your findings and adjust as needed until you create a blend that provides the relief you seek. This exercise helps you discover effective combinations and deepens your understanding of how different oils interact.

## 6.3 STEAM INHALATION METHODS FOR CONGESTION

Imagine a simple, soothing ritual that can ease the discomfort of congestion and bring clarity to your breathing in just minutes. Steam inhalation, a tried-and-true method, offers precisely this kind of relief. Combining the warmth of steam with the therapeutic properties of essential oils can create a natural remedy that helps clear your airways and loosen stubborn mucus. The moisture from the steam softens and thins mucus, making it easier to expel and reducing the pressure in your sinuses. This straightforward method can be done in the comfort of your home, offering a spa-like experience with tangible benefits for your respiratory health.

Bring a pot of water to a gentle boil to perform steam inhalation effectively. Once the water is steaming, remove it from the heat and carefully transfer it to a large, heat-resistant bowl. Add a few drops of your chosen essential oil—usually, three to five drops are sufficient. Tea tree oil is an excellent choice for its antimicrobial properties, which can help fight any lingering pathogens in your airways. Lavender oil, known for its calming effects, can soothe irritated passages while also allowing you to relax. Once the oil is added, lean over the bowl, keeping a safe distance to avoid burns. Drape a towel over your head to create a tent-like enclosure that traps the steam. Please close your eyes, breathe deeply, and allow the aromatic steam to work its magic for about five to ten minutes. This method helps clear your sinuses and offers peace in your busy day.

Safety is paramount when using steam inhalation. Always maintain a safe distance from the hot water to prevent burns. The steam should feel warm and comforting, not scalding. Adjust your position as needed to ensure comfort. It's also important to limit the duration of your steam session. Five to ten minutes is generally enough to achieve benefits without risking overexposure. Prolonged inhalation can lead to dizziness or irritation, so listen to your body and take breaks if needed. If you experience any discomfort or irritation, discontinue the session immediately. Also, be cautious if you have respiratory conditions like asthma, as steam inhalation might trigger symptoms. Consulting a healthcare provider beforehand can help ensure safety.

Choosing suitable essential oils for steam inhalation can enhance the experience and effectiveness. Tea tree oil is particularly beneficial due to its antimicrobial properties. It can help reduce inflammation and fight bacteria, offering a natural way to support your body's defenses against respiratory infections. Lavender oil's soothing effects make it ideal for calming irritated airways and promoting relaxation. Consider experimenting with other oils like chamomile, which offers anti-inflammatory benefits, or rosemary, known for its ability to support respiratory health. Each oil brings unique properties and aromas, allowing you to tailor your steam inhalation to your specific needs and preferences.

Once you've completed your steam inhalation session, take a moment to assess how you feel. This simple practice incorporated into your routine makes breathing easier and your mind clearer. It can provide continuous support for your respiratory system. It's a natural way to manage congestion and promote overall well-being. Whether you're dealing with seasonal allergies, a stubborn cold, or just looking for a way to unwind, steam inhalation with essential oils offers a soothing, effective solution. The warmth of the steam, combined with the healing power of essential oils, transforms your routine into a nurturing ritual that supports both body and mind.

## 6.4 OILS FOR SEASONAL ALLERGIES

As the seasons change, many people find themselves battling allergy symptoms that disrupt their daily lives. Sneezing, itchy eyes, and congestion can make even the simplest tasks feel burdensome. Essential oils offer a natural way to manage these symptoms, providing relief without the side effects often associated with over-the-counter medications. Lavender oil is known for its antihistamine effects, which help to reduce the body's reaction to allergens. By calming the histamine response, lavender can lessen symptoms like sneezing and itching. Its soothing aroma also promotes relaxation, which can be beneficial when allergies leave you feeling run down. Chamomile oil, another effective option, works by reducing inflammation. The anti-inflammatory compounds in chamomile can help ease congestion and soothe irritated nasal passages, offering a gentle way to calm the body's response to allergens.

The mechanisms behind these oils' effectiveness lie in their interaction with the body's immune response. Lavender oil, for instance, contains linalool and linalyl acetate, compounds that have been shown to inhibit the release of histamines. This action helps control the body's allergic response, relieving common symptoms. Chamomile oil, rich in azulene and bisabolol, acts as a natural anti-inflammatory, helping to reduce swelling and irritation. Chamomile can help clear blocked nasal passages and ease breathing by targeting inflammation. These oils address the symptoms and support the body's natural defenses, providing a holistic approach to managing allergies.

Consider incorporating these oils into your daily routine through topical applications and personal inhalers to use these oils for allergy relief effectively. Mixing essential oils with a carrier oil such as coconut or almond oil allows for safe application to the skin. Apply this blend to areas like the chest, temples, or behind the ears to experience the soothing effects. For on-the-go relief, personal inhalers offer a convenient solution. Add a few drops of your chosen oil to a cotton wick inside the inhaler, then inhale deeply when needed. This method provides quick access to the oils' benefits, allowing you to manage symptoms wherever you are.

Real-life experiences attest to the effectiveness of essential oils in managing seasonal allergies. Consider the story of Emily, a frequent allergy sufferer who found herself relying on antihistamines to get through the day. Tired of the drowsiness they caused, she turned to essential oils as an alternative. She discovered a noticeable reduction in her symptoms by using a lavender and chamomile blend in a personal inhaler. The oils helped clear her nasal passages, allowing her to breathe easier and focus on her work. Emily's experience highlights the potential of essential oils to provide relief without unwanted side effects, offering a natural and effective alternative for allergy management.

As we conclude this exploration of essential oils for respiratory health, it's clear that these natural remedies offer a powerful tool for enhancing your well-being. From easing congestion to managing allergy symptoms, essential oils provide versatile solutions that align with your body's natural processes. In the next chapter, we'll focus on how these oils can support digestive health, offering insight into another aspect of holistic wellness.

# MAKE A DIFFERENCE WITH YOUR REVIEW

## UNLOCK THE POWER OF GENEROSITY

***"The smallest act of kindness is worth more than the grandest intention."***

— OSCAR WILDE

People who give without expecting anything in return live happier lives. So, let's make a difference together!

Would you help someone just like you—curious about essential oils but unsure where to start?

My mission is to make using essential oils easy and fun for everyone.

But to reach more people, I need your help.

Most people choose books based on reviews. So, I'm asking you to help a fellow essential oil enthusiast by leaving a review.

It costs nothing and takes less than a minute, but it could change someone's essential oil journey. Your review could help...

- one more small business provides for their community.
- one more entrepreneur supports their family.
- one more client transformed their life.
- one more dream come true.

To make a difference, scan the QR code below and leave a review:

**https://a.co/d/0TyNGze**

If you love helping others, you're my kind of person. Thank you from the bottom of my heart!

*Nina Collins*

# 7

# DIY HOUSEHOLD CLEANING

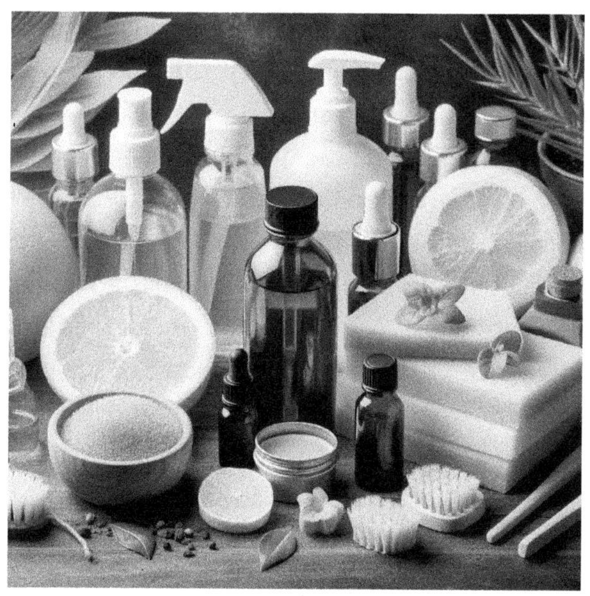

Imagine walking into your home, greeted not by the harsh chemical smell of cleaners but by the fresh, invigorating scent of lemon and eucalyptus. This isn't just a pleasant experience; it's a healthier choice for you and the environment. Essential oils transform cleaning, turning a mundane chore into a sensory delight. They offer a natural alternative to commercial cleaning products that often contain harmful chemicals. You can avoid these harsh substances by using essential oils, which can irritate the skin, eyes, and respiratory system. Essential oils are derived from plants, making them non-toxic and biodegradable, ensuring that your cleaning routine supports a healthy home and planet.

## 7.1 COMBATTING BACTERIA

Natural cleaning sprays are an excellent starting point for incorporating essential oils into your cleaning routine. These sprays are both practical and easy to make. Begin with a basic recipe using a vinegar and water base. Vinegar is a powerful natural disinfectant, quickly cutting through grease and grime. Add lemon essential oil to this mixture. Renowned for its ability to cut through grease, lemon oil leaves surfaces sparkling clean and imparts a fresh, uplifting scent that can boost your mood. Consider adding a few drops of tea tree oil for added antimicrobial properties. Tea tree oil is renowned for combatting bacteria and viruses, providing extra protection against germs. This combination creates a robust all-purpose cleaner that can be used throughout your home, from countertops to bathroom tiles.

Choosing the suitable essential oils for your cleaning needs can enhance the effectiveness of your homemade solutions. Citrus oils like lemon, orange, and grapefruit are particularly effective for dissolving grease and leaving a streak-free shine. These oils are perfect for kitchen surfaces, where grease buildup is common. Eucalyptus oil, with its antibacterial properties, is another excellent choice. It's beneficial for disinfecting surfaces and purifying the air. Eucalyptus oil's refreshing scent also helps clear the mind, making cleaning more enjoyable. These oils clean and leave a lingering freshness, transforming your home into a fragrant sanctuary.

Customizing your cleaning solutions to address specific challenges is easy with essential oils. For instance, if you're dealing with stubborn stains, you might adjust the vinegar concentration in your spray. A higher concentration of vinegar can help tackle tough spots while adding essential oils ensures the solution remains pleasant-smelling. For a refreshing twist, consider adding peppermint oil to your cleaning spray. Its crisp, refreshing aroma freshens the air and provides a natural deodorizing effect, perfect for eliminating unwanted odors. This customization allows you to tailor your cleaning products to fit your unique needs, ensuring your home is clean and inviting.

**Interactive Element: Create Your Custom Cleaning Spray**

Take a moment to identify a cleaning challenge in your home. Is it greasy kitchen counters or musty bathroom tiles? Using the basic vinegar and lemon oil recipe, experiment by adding a secondary oil like tea tree or peppermint. Adjust the vinegar concentration if needed. Record your formula and note its effectiveness. This exercise personalizes your cleaning routine and empowers you to make informed choices about the products you use.

You're choosing a healthier, more sustainable path by embracing essential oils in your cleaning routine. These natural solutions protect your home from harsh chemicals and create an environment that supports your well-being. With essential oils, cleaning becomes an act of care for your space and the planet, offering a fresh perspective on a daily task.

## 7.2 FRESHENING THE AIR: NATURAL DEODORIZERS

Think about the air you breathe indoors. It's not just about temperature or humidity; it's about freshness. The invisible quality of air can profoundly impact your well-being. Many traditional air fresheners mask odors with synthetic fragrances, often laden with chemicals that can irritate your senses and harm the environment. In contrast, essential oils offer a natural alternative, purifying the air while providing therapeutic aromas. Unlike synthetic options, which merely cloak smells, essential oils neutralize them. This means they don't just cover up kitchen smoke or pet odors—they break them down and replace them with delightful, natural scents that uplift your mood and enhance your living space.

Creating natural air fresheners with essential oils is a straightforward process that can transform your environment. One popular option is the gel air freshener, which combines gelatin with essential oils. Begin by dissolving gelatin in hot water, then add a few drops of your chosen essential oil—lemon for a bright, clean scent or cedarwood for a warm, grounding aroma. Once cooled, the gel solidifies, releasing fresh scents gradually. This method is ideal for small spaces like bathrooms or closets, offering a consistent fragrance without overpowering the senses. Another method is the reed diffuser. Mixing essential oils with carrier oil creates a blend that wicks up through the reeds, gently permeating a room. It's a simple, elegant solution that doubles as decor, bringing visual and olfactory beauty to your home.

Essential oils excel in odor neutralization, a critical aspect of maintaining a pleasant indoor atmosphere. Lemon oil, with its crisp and refreshing scent, is particularly effective in kitchens where cooking odors linger. Its natural degreasing properties effectively eliminate last night's dinner smell, leaving only freshness behind. For those damp, musty areas like basements, cedarwood oil is a wise choice. Known for its rich, woody aroma, cedarwood neutralizes odors and discourages mold and mildew growth, adding an extra layer of protection to your home. These oils offer a dual benefit: they refresh the air while addressing the underlying causes of unpleasant smells.

The beauty of essential oils lies in their versatility and potential for customization. You can experiment with different scent combinations to create a signature aroma that reflects your preferences and mood. Perhaps a mix of lavender and citrus appeals to you, providing a calming yet invigorating scent that soothes while energizing. Alternatively, you might enjoy a seasonal blend, such as clove and cinnamon, which evokes warmth and coziness, perfect for cooler months. This personal touch allows you to tailor the atmosphere of your home, making it a sanctuary that feels uniquely yours. Adjusting the proportions of your oils can lead to a more subtle or intense fragrance, depending on your needs and the space you're working with.

**Interactive Element: Design Your Unique Scent Blend**

Take a moment to reflect on the scents that resonate with you. Are there particular aromas that evoke fond memories or feelings of comfort? Use this insight to guide your choice of essential oils—experiment by combining a few drops of different oils in a small bowl. Note how each combination makes you feel and write down your favorite blends. This exercise personalizes your space and enhances your understanding of scent and its impact on your mood and environment.

As you explore these natural solutions, you empower yourself to create a healthier, more inviting living space. Essential oils offer a simple but profound way to enhance air quality, supporting physical health and emotional well-being. Embrace the potential of these natural deodorizers and discover the difference they can make in your home.

## 7.3 ESSENTIAL OILS FOR MOLD AND MILDEW PREVENTION

Mold and mildew are more than unsightly; they pose significant risks to health and home. These fungi thrive in damp environments, often appearing in bathrooms, basements, and kitchens. Their presence can trigger allergic reactions, manifesting as sneezing, itchy eyes, and skin rashes. For those with asthma or other respiratory issues, the spores released by mold can exacerbate symptoms, leading to wheezing and shortness of breath. Beyond health, mold and mildew can damage household surfaces and structures, leading to costly repairs. Given these challenges, prevention is crucial. Essential oils, with their natural antifungal properties, offer an effective way to combat these unwelcome guests.

Tea tree oil stands out for its potent antifungal compounds. Extracted from the leaves of the Melaleuca plant, tea tree oil has long been recognized for its ability to tackle various fungi, including those that cause mold. When used correctly, it can penetrate the cell walls of mold spores, inhibiting their growth and spread. With its robust antimold properties, clove oil pairs perfectly with tea tree oil. Clove oil contains eugenol, a compound that disrupts the cellular processes of mold, making it an effective deterrent. These oils defend against mold and mildew, keeping your home healthier and fresher.

Creating a mold prevention spray is straightforward and requires only a few ingredients. Start with a base of white vinegar, known for its disinfecting properties. Vinegar can kill mold spores on contact, making it an excellent foundation for your spray. Add ten drops of tea tree oil and ten drops of clove oil. Each oil has unique strengths that combine to form a powerful antifungal solution. Mix these ingredients in a spray bottle, shaking well to ensure even distribution. This mixture can be stored and used as needed, making it a convenient addition to your cleaning arsenal. While strong, the natural aroma of these oils dissipates quickly, leaving behind a clean scent.

Applying these solutions effectively is critical to preventing mold growth. Focus on moisture-prone areas such as bathrooms, where steam from showers can create a perfect environment for mold. Regular application is essential; aim to spray these areas once a week or after heavy use. In kitchens, pay attention to areas around sinks and under cabinets, where leaks might occur unnoticed. Using a spray bottle makes application quick and easy, allowing you to cover large areas or precisely target specific spots. Ensure the area is well-ventilated to allow for even drying, reducing the chance of moisture buildup.

Prevention also involves addressing the root causes of mold growth. Keep humidity levels in check by using dehumidifiers in damp areas. Ensure proper ventilation by using exhaust fans in kitchens and bathrooms, especially during and after cooking or showering. Regularly inspect your home for leaks or water damage, addressing any issues promptly. Combining these preventative measures with the power of essential oils creates a robust strategy for keeping mold at bay. This approach preserves the integrity of your home and safeguards the health of everyone who lives there.

## 7.4 DIY DISH AND LAUNDRY DETERGENTS

Imagine a world where you control what goes into your daily products, from dish soap to laundry detergent. The idea of homemade detergents isn't just about creativity; it's about empowerment and safety. Making your cleaning products offers numerous benefits, including cost savings and the ability to customize formulas to meet specific needs. Store-bought detergents often contain harsh chemicals that irritate skin or harm the environment. By crafting your own, you ensure that what touches your dishes and clothes is gentle, effective, and environmentally friendly.

To create a natural dish detergent, start with a castile soap base, a versatile and biodegradable soap derived from vegetable oils. Its mild nature makes it perfect for cleaning without leaving harmful residues. Add a few drops of lemon essential oil, known for its grease-cutting ability and fresh scent, to enhance the cleaning power. Rosemary oil complements this by offering natural antibacterial properties, ensuring your dishes come out clean and sanitized. This combination creates a potent yet gentle cleaner that leaves your dishes sparkling and your kitchen smelling delightful. Mix these ingredients in a bottle, shake well, and store them conveniently for easy access during dishwashing.

Laundry routines also benefit from including essential oils, which add fragrance and antimicrobial properties to your wash. Lavender oil is a classic choice for bedding and linens, infusing them with a calming scent that can promote relaxation and restful sleep. Its natural antibacterial qualities also help keep your sheets fresh and clean. Eucalyptus oil is ideal for gym clothes, which often harbor strong odors. Known for its refreshing aroma and disinfecting power, eucalyptus oil helps to eliminate odors and bacteria, leaving your workout gear fresh and ready for the next session. These oils enhance the cleaning process and make laundry a more enjoyable chore by filling your space with pleasant aromas.

A simple recipe for DIY laundry detergent involves a few common household ingredients. Combine baking soda and washing soda, natural cleaning agents that help soften water and break down dirt and grease. Grate a bar of unscented soap, such as castile, and mix it with the sodas. Add several drops of essential oils, like lavender or eucalyptus, to impart fragrance and additional cleaning power. This mixture creates a gentle yet effective detergent that cleans thoroughly without the harshness of commercial products. It's safe for all fabrics and works well in standard and high-efficiency washing machines.

Enhancing laundry freshness can be as simple as adding a few drops of essential oil to wool dryer balls. These balls help to soften clothes naturally while reducing drying time. The addition of essential oils infuses your laundry with a lasting scent that can be tailored to your preferences. You can also create sachets using dried herbs and a few drops of essential oil, placing them in your closets or drawers to keep clothes smelling fresh. These natural alternatives provide a chemical-free way to maintain fresh-smelling laundry and offer an opportunity to personalize the fragrance to suit your taste.

Making your own dish and laundry detergents ensures a safer environment for your family and contributes to a more sustainable world. These homemade solutions eliminate the need for plastic containers and reduce the overall chemical footprint in your home. Essential oils bring the added benefit of aromatherapy, turning mundane tasks into moments of sensory pleasure. Through these practices, you align daily chores with a commitment to health and sustainability, paving the way for a cleaner, greener household.

# 8

# PERSONAL CARE AND BEAUTY

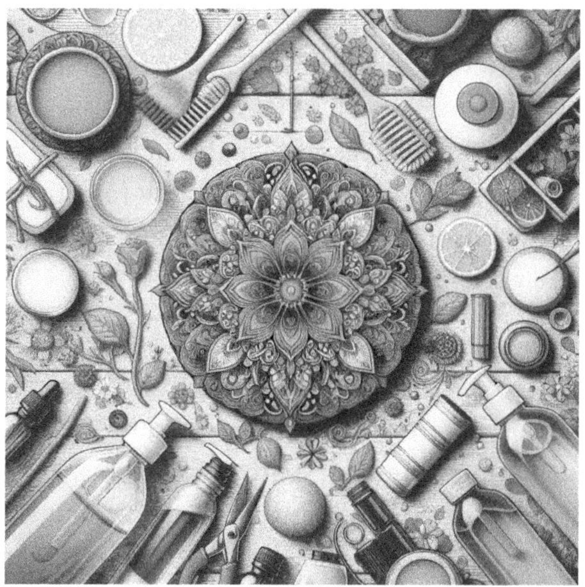

Imagine standing in front of your bathroom mirror, surveying an array of skincare products that promise the world but deliver little more than frustration. The quest for clear, radiant skin can feel like a daunting journey. Yet, a natural, effective path has been embraced for centuries: essential oils. These potent plant extracts offer solutions for common skin concerns like acne, dryness, and aging. You can tap into nature's bounty to transform your skin by incorporating them into your skincare routine.

## 8.1 SKINCARE BASICS WITH ESSENTIAL OILS

Essential oils hold a wealth of benefits for skincare. For those struggling with acne, tea tree oil is a game-changer. Tea tree oil is known for its antimicrobial and anti-inflammatory properties, which help combat acne-causing bacteria such as Cutibacterium acnes—reducing breakouts and soothing inflamed skin. Its effectiveness is well-documented, offering a natural alternative to harsher treatments (Source 1). Meanwhile, rosehip oil shines as an anti-aging powerhouse. Rich in vitamins A and C, it aids in reducing fine lines and promoting a youthful glow. Its ability to penetrate deep into the skin ensures that its nourishing benefits are delivered where needed most.

Understanding your skin type is crucial when selecting suitable oils. For oily skin, jojoba oil is an excellent choice. Its structure closely resembles the skin's natural sebum, helping to balance oil production without clogging pores. This makes it ideal for controlling shine and keeping skin clear. On the other hand, if your skin tends to be dry, argan oil can provide the hydration it craves. Argan oil is rich in essential fatty acids and antioxidants, providing deep moisturization while protecting the skin from environmental damage. This dual action makes it a valuable addition for anyone needing extra nourishment.

Creating your skincare products with essential oils can be both satisfying and effective. Consider starting with a soothing toner from aloe vera gel and lavender oil. Aloe vera's hydrating properties, combined with lavender's calming scent and antibacterial benefits, make this toner perfect for refreshing your skin after cleansing. Mix a tablespoon of aloe vera gel with a few drops of lavender oil and apply gently with a cotton pad. A DIY facial serum with frankincense and rose oils can work wonders for a more intensive treatment. Both oils are celebrated for their ability to rejuvenate and revitalize the skin. Combine them with a carrier oil like jojoba for a light, non-greasy serum that absorbs quickly, delivering nutrients and antioxidants directly to your skin.

Incorporating essential oils into your existing skincare routine doesn't have to be complicated. A simple way to start is by adding a few drops of your chosen essential oil to your current moisturizer. This can enhance its effectiveness, providing additional benefits tailored to your skin's needs. For an indulgent treat, try facial steaming with essential oils. Add a drop or two of lavender or chamomile oil to a bowl of hot water, then lean over with a towel over your head to trap the steam. This opens your pores, allowing the oils to penetrate more deeply, and provides a relaxing, spa-like experience.

**Interactive Element: Skincare Reflection**

Consider the current state of your skin and identify any concerns you wish to address. Reflect on your skin type and which essential oils might best support your skincare goals.

Create a simple plan to incorporate one new essential oil into your routine this week and observe how your skin responds. Record your observations and any changes in a journal.

Integrating essential oils into your skincare regimen harnesses nature's power to nurture and protect your skin. These oils offer a versatile, customizable approach to beauty, allowing you to tailor your routine to suit your needs. Embrace the opportunity to explore these natural remedies and discover the radiant, healthy skin that awaits.

## 8.2 CRAFTING CUSTOM PERFUMES AND SCENTS

Imagine stepping into a world where every scent tells a story, a personal narrative crafted by you. That's the magic of natural perfumery. It's not just about smelling good; it's about creating a signature fragrance that reflects who you are. The process begins with understanding the structure of scents like musical chords. Each blend consists of top, middle, and base notes, each playing a role in the fragrance's evolution. Top notes are the first impression, often bright and lively, like a burst of citrus. They catch attention but evaporate quickly. Middle or heart notes provide the fragrance's core, adding depth and character with floral or herbal tones. Finally, base notes are the foundation, the lingering warmth of wood or spices that ground the scent and give it lasting power.

Creating your own perfume blend involves balancing these notes to achieve harmony. Start by selecting oils from different categories—floral, citrus, and woodsy are a classic combination. For a balanced blend, consider the 30:50:20

ratio: 30% top notes, 50% middle notes, and 20% base notes. Begin with a citrus-like orange for the top note. Its vibrant, zesty aroma uplifts and energizes. For the middle note, jasmine offers a sweet, intoxicating scent that adds elegance and complexity. As for the base, sandalwood provides a creamy, woody undertone that complements and anchors the lighter notes. Mix ten drops of each essential oil in a small glass bottle, allowing the blend to sit for a day to harmonize fully.

Let's explore signature recipes you can try. The "Citrus Spice" blend combines orange, clove, and sandalwood. Orange offers a refreshing start, clove adds a warm, spicy twist, and sandalwood rounds it out with its rich, grounding presence. This blend is perfect for those who enjoy vibrant yet cozy scents. On the other hand, the "Floral Dream" blend features jasmine, bergamot, and patchouli. Jasmine's floral sweetness is complemented by bergamot's fresh, citrusy zest, with patchouli adding a deep, earthy finish. This blend is ideal for a more romantic, sophisticated fragrance.

Once you've crafted your blend, consider how you'll wear it. Roll-on perfumes are a convenient option and easy to apply and carry. Dilute your mixture with a carrier oil like jojoba or sweet almond, fill a rollerball bottle, and apply to pulse points such as wrists and neck. This method provides a personal scent experience that evolves throughout the day. For a more traditional approach, solid perfumes are another option. Create a base with beeswax and carrier oil, melt them together, and stir in your essential oil blend. Pour the mixture into small tins and let it solidify. These practical and travel-friendly solid perfumes offer a subtle, long-lasting fragrance.

Crafting custom perfumes allows you to express your individuality. Each blend reflects your mood, style, and preferences. The possibilities are endless, limited only by your imagination. You'll discover scents that resonate with you as you experiment with different combinations, offering a genuinely personalized fragrance experience.

## 8.3 HAIR CARE SOLUTIONS WITH NATURAL OILS

Imagine running your fingers through hair that feels vibrant and healthy, each strand reflecting the care you've put into it. Essential oils offer a natural approach to achieving this, addressing common hair concerns like dandruff, dryness, and lack of shine. Rosemary oil is particularly renowned for its role in stimulating hair growth. Its ability to promote cellular generation is a valuable ally in enhancing hair thickness and health. When massaged into the scalp, rosemary oil can boost blood circulation, which helps deliver nutrients to hair follicles, encouraging growth and vitality. With its refreshing menthol content, peppermint oil offers similar benefits by invigorating the scalp and promoting a healthy environment for hair growth. Its cooling effect can soothe irritation and reduce dandruff, making it an excellent choice for maintaining scalp health.

Creating your hair care products with essential oils can be simple and rewarding. Consider a DIY dry shampoo using lavender oil and cornstarch. This combo absorbs excess oil and leaves a gentle fragrance that refreshes your hair between washes. Mix equal parts of cornstarch and baking soda, then add a few drops of lavender oil. Apply a makeup brush to your roots, comb through them, and enjoy the fresh feeling. A hair mask made from coconut oil and ylang-ylang can work wonders for deeper nourishment. Coconut oil's moisturizing properties penetrate the hair shaft, while ylang-ylang adds a touch of luxury with its floral scent. Combine a tablespoon of coconut oil with a few drops of ylang-ylang, warm the mixture slightly, and apply it to your hair, focusing on the ends. Leave it on for about 30 minutes before rinsing thoroughly for soft, lustrous locks.

Carrier oils play a crucial role in enhancing the effectiveness of essential oils in hair care. Argan oil, often hailed as "liquid gold," is a superb moisturizer that adds shine and softness without weighing hair down. Its high vitamin E and fatty acids make it perfect for repairing and nourishing dry, damaged hair. Similarly, castor oil is celebrated for its ability to strengthen hair, thanks to its rich ricinoleic acid content. It can fortify hair strands, reduce breakage, and promote fuller, thicker hair growth. When used as a carrier, these oils allow essential oils to be spread evenly across the hair and scalp, maximizing their benefits and ensuring a gentle, non-irritating application.

Incorporating essential oils into your daily hairstyling routine can add a touch of nature's luxury. Add a few drops of your favorite essential oil to styling gels or sprays. This imparts a pleasant scent and provides additional nourishment and protection. Try a hot oil treatment with essential oils for a more profound treatment. Heat a mixture of your chosen carrier oil and essential oils, apply it to your hair, and cover it with a warm towel for about 20 minutes. This process helps seal moisture into your hair, leaving it silky and manageable. It's a delightful way to indulge your hair in a spa-like experience right at home.

Experimenting with essential oils in hair care opens a world of possibilities. You'll discover what works best for your hair type and concerns as you explore different combinations and applications. The flexibility of these natural ingredients allows you to customize your hair care routine, providing solutions that are as unique as you are. With each application, you're not just treating your hair—nurturing it with the best nature offers.

## 8.4 DIY LIP BALMS AND BODY BUTTER

Imagine creating your own lip balms and body butter, perfectly tailored to your tastes and needs. The appeal of homemade products lies in their customization and the purity of ingredients used. When you make your own, you sidestep synthetic additives often found in commercial products, instead embracing nature's ingredients' simplicity and effectiveness. This means avoiding unnecessary chemicals and nourishing your skin with wholesome elements. Moreover, crafting these items at home allows you to experiment with scents and textures, creating a product that's uniquely yours.

Crafting lip balm is a straightforward process that yields satisfying results. Begin with a blend of beeswax, coconut oil, and peppermint essential oil. Beeswax is a protective barrier that locks in moisture and provides a smooth application. Coconut oil is renowned for its moisturizing properties, keeping your lips soft and hydrated. Peppermint essential oil adds a refreshing tingle and offers antimicrobial benefits. To make your lip balm, melt 1 part beeswax and 1 part coconut oil in a double boiler. Once melted, remove from heat and stir in a few drops of peppermint oil. Pour the mixture into small containers and let it solidify. The result is a nourishing balm that leaves your lips feeling rejuvenated and fresh.

Creating rich body butter is equally rewarding, offering a luxurious treat for your skin. Combining shea butter, cocoa butter, and vanilla essential oil makes an indulgent moisturizer that hydrates and protects. Shea butter is rich in vitamins and fatty acids, deeply nourishing the skin and promoting elasticity. Cocoa butter adds a creamy texture with its high antioxidant content, helping to repair and protect the skin. Vanilla essential oil lends a comforting aroma, turning each application into a sensory delight. To make this body butter, gently melt two parts shea butter and 1 part cocoa butter, then cool them slightly before whipping them with an electric mixer. Add a few drops of vanilla oil as the mixture thickens and continue beating until light and fluffy. Store in a jar, ready to soothe and hydrate your skin whenever needed.

These recipes are just starting points. Part of the fun of making your own products is the ability to experiment with different ingredients and essential oils. Adjusting the ratio of butter to oils can alter the consistency you like—more shea butter for a firmer feel or more cocoa butter for a smoother, silkier texture. You might also incorporate calming essential oils like lavender or chamomile to add soothing effects, perfect for nighttime relaxation. Experimenting with combinations allows you to discover what works best for your skin and preferences, making the process as enjoyable as the product.

Beyond the practical benefits, crafting your own lip balms and body butter is an exercise in creativity and mindfulness. It encourages you to engage with natural ingredients and explore their potential, deepening your connection to the products you use daily. The satisfaction of using something you've made with your own hands, knowing every ingredient and its purpose, is gratifying. These personalized creations make thoughtful gifts, offering a touch of handmade care that friends and family will appreciate.

As you explore these DIY projects, remember that the journey is as valuable as the destination. Each experiment is an opportunity to learn and grow, to fine-tune your skills and preferences. Embrace the process and enjoy the discovery of what these natural elements can do for your skin. In the next chapter, we'll explore how essential oils can be incorporated into your kitchen and culinary practices, extending their benefits beyond personal care and daily nourishment.

9

# KITCHEN AND CULINARY USES

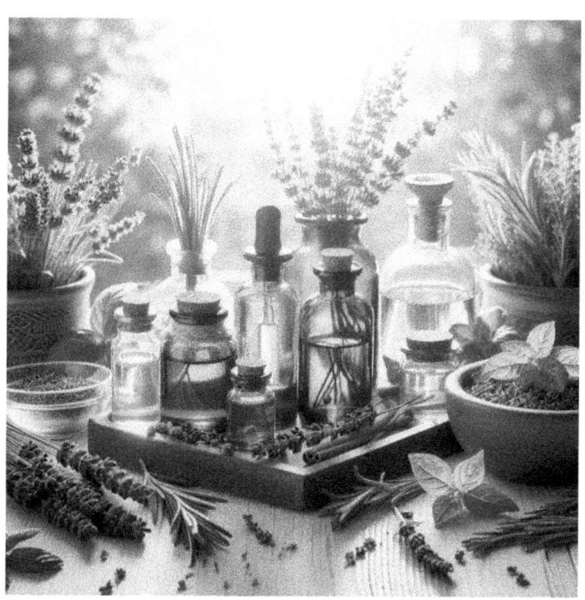

Imagine walking into your kitchen, where the scent of fresh lemons and mint fills the air. It's not just any day; you're about to explore a new culinary adventure with essential oils. These oils, extracted from the purest parts of plants, can transform your cooking experience. They offer a depth of flavor that is both surprising and delightful. However, as with any powerful ingredient, using essential oils in food requires a careful approach. Their potency demands respect and understanding to ensure your dishes remain safe and delectable.

## 9.1 FOOD-GRADE ESSENTIAL OILS

When you incorporate essential oils into your cooking, the first step is recognizing which oils are suitable for culinary use. Not all essential oils are created equal, and "food-grade" is a term that lacks legal recognition, but hints at oils intended for safe consumption when used correctly. The F.D.A. categorizes some essential oils as Generally Recognized As Safe (G.R.A.S.) for specific culinary purposes. These include citrus oils like lemon and orange, which can add a vibrant zest to your dishes, and peppermint, known for its refreshing kick. However, oils such as wintergreen and eucalyptus should be avoided in the kitchen, as their ingestion can pose health risks.

Understanding the potency of essential oils is crucial. These are concentrated substances, and a little goes a long way. Understanding the importance of dilution in recipes is vital when using certain ingredients. Mixing essential oils with carrier oils such as olive or coconut oil can help disperse their intense flavors. This method tempers the intensity and ensures an even distribution throughout your dish. Another effective technique is using sugar or salt as a dispersing medium. By blending a drop of essential oil with a pinch of sugar or salt, you can create a flavorful base that infuses your dish with subtlety. This approach works well in sweet and savory recipes, allowing you to experiment without overpowering the palate.

Accurate measurement is another integral part of cooking with essential oils. Given their strength, even a single drop can make a significant impact. Using droppers can help achieve precision, preventing any accidental overuse. Start with one drop and taste as you go, adjusting to meet your preferences. This method ensures that the oils enhance your dish rather than dominate it, allowing the natural flavors of other ingredients to shine through. Balance is essential in culinary applications, and essential oils are no exception. Their role is to complement, not overpower, the existing flavors in your dish.

**Interactive Element: Essential Oil Cooking Checklist**

- Choose Wisely: Select only food-grade essential oils. Start with lemon, orange, or peppermint.
- Dilution First: Mix oils with olive or coconut oil for even distribution. Consider using sugar or salt for added control.
- Measure Precisely: Use droppers for exact measurements. Begin with one drop and adjust to taste.
- Avoid Overpowering: Test flavors gradually. Focus on balance within the dish.

By embracing these guidelines, you can unlock the unique potential of essential oils in your cooking. They offer not just flavor but also a way to engage with the essence of plants in a new, meaningful way. As you stand in your kitchen with a dropper in hand, you're not just cooking—you're crafting an experience that connects you to the essence of nature's bounty.

## 9.2 FLAVORING BEVERAGES AND DESSERTS

Imagine sipping a chilled glass of iced tea on a warm afternoon, the subtle notes of lemon and lavender dancing on your palate. Essential oils can transform beverages and desserts, infusing them with vibrant flavors that elevate the ordinary to the extraordinary. Like lemon and orange, Citrus oils bring bright and refreshing accents to drinks, making them perfect for hot summer days. Meanwhile, floral oils such as lavender and rose add a delicate, aromatic touch to desserts, creating an experience that is both sensory and indulgent. These oils open possibilities, allowing you to experiment and craft unique culinary delights.

Take, for instance, a refreshing lemon and lavender iced tea. Begin by brewing your favorite black or green tea, then add a few drops of lemon essential oil for a zesty kick. Stir in a drop of lavender oil, introducing a fragrant note that complements the citrus perfectly. Allow the tea to cool before pouring it over ice, garnishing it with a slice of lemon or a sprig of fresh lavender. This drink not only refreshes but also uplifts the spirit, offering a moment of calm during a busy day. Another delightful option is an orange and mint-infused sparkling water. Add a drop of orange oil and a hint of peppermint to a glass of chilled sparkling water. The result is a crisp, invigorating beverage that tantalizes the taste buds and refreshes the body.

In desserts, essential oils can infuse your creations with layers of flavor that surprise and delight. Consider a rich chocolate ganache, where peppermint oil can transform it into a cool, refreshing treat. Melt your chocolate and cream together, then stir in the peppermint oil. This addition enhances the richness of the chocolate and adds a cooling contrast that enlivens the dessert. Similarly, vanilla essential oil can elevate your frosting or cake batter. A few drops of this oil can intensify the vanilla flavor, making your baked goods irresistibly aromatic and flavorful. The key is to blend the oils smoothly, allowing them to integrate fully without overpowering the other ingredients.

Encouraging creativity in the kitchen is part of the joy of using essential oils. Imagine combining citrus and spice oils to create holiday cookies with warmth and zest. A few drops of orange oil, paired with a hint of cinnamon or clove, can evoke the cozy flavors of the season in each bite. Or picture a custard infused with essential oils, where the creaminess of the dessert is complemented by a gentle floral or citrus note. The possibilities are endless, whether it's a hint of lavender in your vanilla custard or a touch of lime in a coconut cream. These oils invite you to explore and create flavors that are uniquely yours, encouraging a culinary adventure that is both fun and rewarding.

Experiment with different combinations to find what resonates with your taste buds. Essential oils offer a palette of flavors that can transform the mundane into the memorable. By blending, tasting, and adjusting, you can discover new favorites and signature creations that reflect your personal style. This process invites you to engage with your food more deeply, exploring the nuances of flavor and aroma that these potent oils provide. As you experiment, you'll find that the kitchen becomes not just a place of routine but a space of creativity and expression.

## 9.3 INFUSING OILS INTO SAVORY DISHES

Imagine the aroma of a kitchen filled with the scent of rosemary and thyme, mingling as they enhance the flavors of a roasted chicken. Essential oils can transform your savory dishes, offering a depth of flavor that dried herbs alone cannot achieve. These concentrated oils capture the essence of fresh herbs and spices, providing a vibrant boost to your culinary creations. Herbaceous oils like rosemary and thyme are perfect for marinades and dressings, infusing dishes with a robust, earthy quality. Meanwhile, spicy oils such as black pepper and basil can elevate meats and vegetables, adding a layer of complexity that tantalizes the taste buds.

Consider a rosemary and thyme-infused roasted chicken. Begin by creating a marinade with olive oil, a splash of white wine, and a drop each of rosemary and thyme essential oils. The oils will impart their distinctive flavors into the meat, enhancing the natural richness of the chicken. Allow the chicken to marinate for a few hours, letting the flavors meld. The aroma will fill your kitchen as it roasts, promising a comforting and flavorful meal.

Likewise, adding garlic and basil oils can enhance a pasta sauce. Sauté garlic in olive oil, then add a few drops of garlic essential oil to intensify the flavor. Stir in crushed tomatoes and a drop of basil oil, allowing the sauce to simmer until it reaches the desired consistency. The result is a sauce that bursts with the freshness of summer, even in the depths of winter.

Balancing flavors when using essential oils is crucial. Their potency requires a thoughtful approach to ensure that they complement rather than overpower other ingredients. Start with a small amount, allowing the oils to enhance rather than dominate. Taste frequently, adjusting the quantities to suit your preference. The goal is to achieve harmony in your dish, where each flavor is distinct yet integrated. For instance, pair bold oils like oregano or clove with milder counterparts like lemon or parsley to create a balanced profile. This interplay of flavors can elevate a simple dish to something extraordinary, showcasing the versatility of essential oils in savory cooking.

Marinating and seasoning with essential oils offers another avenue for culinary exploration. Consider combining your chosen oils with vinegar or wine when preparing a marinade. This helps to dilute the oils and adds another layer of flavor. A red wine vinegar with a touch of oregano oil can create a robust marinade for lamb, while a white wine and lemon oil combination can brighten seafood dishes. For grilling, incorporate essential oils into your spice blends. Mixing cumin, paprika, and a drop of black pepper oil can add a smoky depth to grilled vegetables. The key is to experiment with different combinations, discovering what enhances the natural flavors of your ingredients.

The world of savory cooking with essential oils is vast and inviting. Each oil offers a unique profile that can unexpectedly enhance your dishes. Understanding how to balance these potent flavors opens the door to a new level of culinary creativity. The possibilities are endless, limited only by your imagination and willingness to explore. As you experiment, you'll find that essential oils can become an integral part of your savory cooking repertoire, transforming everyday meals into gourmet experiences.

## 9.4 CREATING HERBAL VINEGARS AND DRESSINGS

Imagine transforming a simple salad into a gourmet experience with just a splash of homemade herbal vinegar. Essential oils can elevate your culinary creations by enhancing acidity and adding layers of flavor that are both complex and delightful. Crafting herbal vinegar with essential oils brings subtle complexities to your dishes and offers an aromatic twist that redefines your approach to condiments. The process begins with understanding how these oils can interact with vinegars to create a symphony of taste. For instance, combining balsamic vinegar with a few drops of oregano and thyme oils can infuse a rich, earthy aroma that complements robust salads or grilled vegetables. The rich and tangy balsamic flavor complements the herbal notes, resulting in a versatile and flavorful vinegar.

To craft this herbal vinegar:

1. Start by selecting a high-quality balsamic vinegar as your base.
2. Pour it into a sterilized glass bottle, leaving some space at the top.
3. Add a few drops of oregano and thyme essential oils.

4. Shake the bottle gently to blend the ingredients, then let the mixture sit for a few days in a cool, dark place to allow the flavors to meld.

The importance of the resting period cannot be overstated, as it allows the essential oils to fully permeate the vinegar, imbuing it with their distinctive aromatic qualities. This process is what transforms the mixture into a sophisticated condiment, capable of elevating a wide range of dishes. Its versatility shines when added to salads, infusing them with nuanced flavors, or used in marinades to tenderize and enhance the taste of meats. Drizzled over roasted meats, this herbal vinegar introduces an extra dimension of flavor, turning simple meals into culinary delights. The careful melding of the oils' essence with the vinegar results in a creation far greater than the sum of its parts, offering a simple way to bring a gourmet touch to everyday cooking.

Consider crafting a white wine vinegar infused with dill and lemon oils for a lighter option. The crisp acidity of white wine vinegar provides a perfect canvas for the bright, refreshing notes of lemon oil, while the dill adds a hint of herbal sophistication. This combination is particularly well-suited for seafood dishes or light, summery salads. To prepare this infusion, follow the same steps as balsamic vinegar, adjusting the oil ratios to taste. The finished product is a delicate, aromatic vinegar that adds a touch of elegance to any dish.

In addition to vinegar, essential oils can create distinctive and flavorful dressings. For example, a lemon and basil vinaigrette can bring brightness to salads and grilled vegetables. Start by whisking together olive oil, a splash of white wine vinegar, and a few drops of lemon and basil oil. Adjust the seasoning with salt and pepper to taste. This simple yet sophisticated dressing highlights the ingredients' natural flavors, making it a versatile addition to your culinary repertoire.

Try a creamy avocado dressing enhanced with lime oil for a creamier alternative. Blend ripe avocados with Greek yogurt, a hint of garlic, and a few drops of lime essential oil. The result is a rich, tangy dressing that pairs beautifully with tacos, sandwiches, or as a dip for fresh vegetables. This dressing provides a creamy texture and a refreshing zing that can enhance any meal.

Encouraging experimentation with these condiments can lead to endless culinary possibilities. Mix essential oils with mustard or honey to create sweet and tangy dressings. The interplay of citrus oils with fresh herbs can create a balanced profile that complements a variety of dishes. For instance, pairing orange oil with rosemary in a honey mustard dressing can add a delightful twist to your salad. These combinations invite creativity and personal expression, allowing you to craft condiments that reflect your unique taste preferences.

You can discover new favorites and expand your culinary horizons by exploring different flavor pairings. Essential oils offer a world of flavors waiting to be unlocked; each drops a gateway to a new experience. As you experiment, you'll find that these oils can elevate your cooking, transforming everyday meals into extraordinary feasts. With a willingness to explore and a few essential oils on hand, your kitchen's possibilities are endless.

# 10

# EMOTIONAL AND MENTAL WELL-BEING

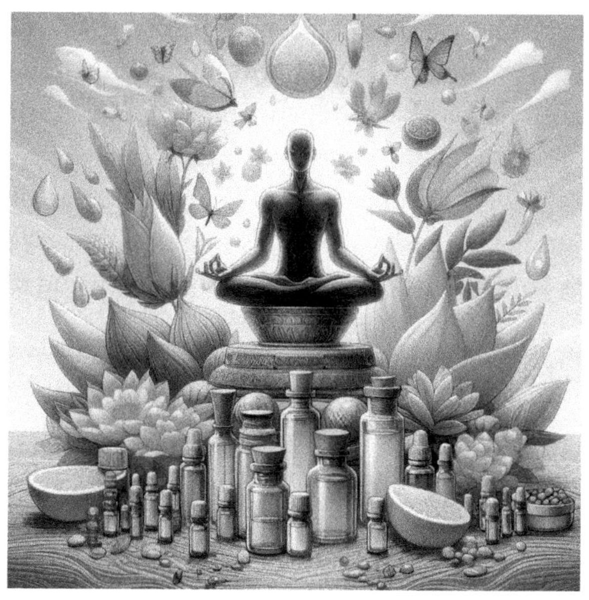

Imagine sitting at your desk, papers scattered, a deadline looming. Your mind feels like a jumbled mess, unable to focus. This is a familiar scene for many. The demands of modern life often leave you searching for clarity and concentration. With their potent aromas, essential oils naturally sharpen your mind and help you find focus amidst chaos. This chapter explores how you can incorporate these age-old remedies to enhance mental clarity and productivity.

## 10.1 OILS FOR FOCUS AND CONCENTRATION

Regarding mental clarity, few oils match the prowess of rosemary and peppermint. These oils are known for their refreshing properties and have been used for a long time to stimulate the mind and enhance concentration. Rosemary oil stands out for its cognitive benefits. Research highlights its potential to improve memory retention, thanks to active ingredients like carnosic acid and rosmarinic acid. These compounds are believed to support mental function through antioxidant, neuroprotective, and anti-inflammatory actions (Source 1). Imagine the refreshing scent of rosemary wafting through the air, its aroma waking your senses and preparing your brain for the tasks ahead. It's more than just a pleasant smell; it's your ally in keeping your mind sharp and focused.

With its crisp, clean aroma, peppermint oil is another powerhouse for mental alertness. The invigorating scent of peppermint stimulates your senses, promoting wakefulness and attentiveness. It's like a brisk walk in the cool morning air, clearing the fog from your mind. Peppermint oil is believed to enhance cognitive performance by increasing oxygen levels in the brain, improving alertness, and reducing fatigue. When the midday slump hits, a whiff of peppermint can be the natural pick-me-up you need.

Incorporating these oils into your daily routine can be both simple and effective. Consider diffusing peppermint oil during study sessions. The steady release of its aroma can help maintain your focus and keep distractions at bay. Alternatively, apply diluted rosemary oil to your temples before diving into work. The direct application allows the oil to interact with your skin and senses, offering a gentle yet persistent boost to your concentration. This method involves inhaling the scent and creating a ritual that signals your brain to switch to focus mode.

Crafting a focused environment goes beyond just using essential oils. Think about your workspace. Is it conducive to concentration? Combining the use of essential oils with strategic lighting and sound can create a multi-sensory experience that enhances focus. Use focused lighting—such as a desk lamp with an adjustable arm—to illuminate your work area. Pair this with noise-cancelling headphones to block out distractions. Together, these elements create a cocoon of concentration, allowing you to immerse yourself fully in your tasks.

Desk diffusers can be essential for helping maintain focus throughout the day. Opt for a diffuser with intermittent settings, allowing aroma bursts to refresh your mind periodically without overwhelming your senses. This approach helps sustain mental alertness, offering gentle reminders to stay on track. Picture yourself in a workspace where every breath is a prompt to focus, where the air itself encourages productivity.

### Interactive Element: Create Your Focus Blend

Dive into the art of blending by crafting your very own focus-enhancing elixir. Begin with a foundation of peppermint and rosemary oils, celebrated for their invigorating properties that awaken the mind and sharpen focus. Introduce a dash of lemon oil to infuse the blend with a layer of brightness, its citrus notes cutting through mental fog with ease. Complement this with a drop of cedarwood oil, grounding the blend with its earthy tones and creating a balanced, harmonious aura conducive to concentration. Experiment with varying proportions of these oils to tailor the blend to your personal preference and sensitivity. Perhaps a more pronounced citrus note uplifts your spirits, or maybe a stronger presence of rosemary invigorates your cognitive processes. The journey of discovering the perfect balance for your needs is both an art and a science, offering a deeper connection to the natural world and its bountiful resources. Utilize this personalized blend in a diffuser to envelop your workspace in an aroma that signals your brain to focus, transforming your environment into a haven of productivity. Alternatively, for a more direct and intimate experience, prepare a personal inhaler for use during intense work sessions or moments when concentration wanes. This method provides a quick, potent burst of clarity, immediately re-aligning your senses and mental faculties toward the task at hand. As you integrate these practices into your daily routine, you'll discover the profound impact essential oils can have beyond merely pleasing the senses. They emerge as invaluable allies in your quest for mental clarity, equipping you with natural, effective tools to navigate the complexities and demands of modern life. With each inhalation, you're not just breathing in a fragrance; you're inhaling focus, grounding, and a renewed sense of purpose, all crafted by your own hands.

## 10.2 UPLIFTING SCENTS FOR MOOD ENHANCEMENT

Imagine waking up to the refreshing scent of citrus, a burst of sunshine captured in a bottle. These oils, particularly orange and grapefruit, carry an energizing essence that can transform a mundane morning into a vibrant start. Their zesty aroma does more than please the senses; it elevates the spirit, providing a natural boost to your mood. Citrus oils are renowned for this effect, offering a fresh, lively fragrance that can cut through mental fog and spark joy. They act as a gentle nudge, propelling you into the day with positivity and energy.

Bergamot oil uniquely blends citrus and floral notes, enhancing the mood. It's like a warm embrace, soothing and uplifting simultaneously. Bergamot is particularly noted for its ability to reduce stress, making it a valuable ally in maintaining emotional balance. The key is its connection with the brain's limbic system, which plays a crucial role in emotions and memory. By influencing this system, bergamot can help regulate mood, ease feelings of anxiety, and promote a sense of well-being. Its scent is complex yet comforting, a reminder that nature holds powerful tools for emotional support.

The impact of scent on your emotional state is profound. Aromatic compounds in essential oils can evoke memories and emotions thanks to their interaction with the limbic system. This part of the brain is a direct pathway to your feelings, explaining why certain scents can instantly uplift your mood or transport you to a calm place. When you inhale these aromatic compounds, they travel to the brain, influencing the production of neurotransmitters like serotonin and dopamine—chemicals that play a crucial role in mood regulation. This biochemical response is why a simple scent can trigger powerful emotional changes, brightening a gloomy day.

Creating mood-boosting blends with essential oils can be a delightful exercise in personal well-being. Consider crafting a "Sunny Day" blend, combining sweet orange, lemon, and ylang-ylang. Sweet orange contributes its lively, cheerful aroma, while lemon adds a clean, refreshing note. Ylang-ylang, with its exotic, floral scent, brings a touch of luxury and balance, rounding out the blend beautifully. Use this combination in a diffuser to fill your space with positivity or apply it to pulse points for a personal pick-me-up. Blending these oils becomes a ritual of self-care, a moment to pause and cultivate joy.

Incorporating uplifting oils into your daily routine is a simple yet effective way to maintain a positive mood. Start your day by adding a few drops of citrus oil to your morning shower or skincare routine. The refreshing scent will help you wake up and set a positive tone for the day. As you move through your day, consider using a portable diffuser in personal spaces like your car or workspace. These small devices can release mood-enhancing aromas, providing a boost whenever needed. The subtle presence of these scents constantly reminds you of the natural support available to you.

**Reflection Section: Scent and Memory**

Take a moment to reflect on scents that evoke positive memories or emotions. Consider how you can incorporate these into your daily life. Is there a particular oil that reminds you of a happy time? Use this oil in a diffuser or personal blend and observe how it influences your mood throughout the day. Keep a journal to note any changes or insights, deepening your understanding of how scent impacts your emotional well-being.

## 10.3 COMBATING ANXIETY AND DEPRESSION

In the quiet moments when anxiety starts to creep in or during those days when a cloud of low mood won't lift, essential oils can offer a gentle form of support. Two oils have gained recognition for their calming and mood-stabilizing properties: lavender and clary sage. These oils don't just mask feelings; they interact with your body on a biochemical level to help ease symptoms of anxiety and depression. Lavender oil, known for its soothing floral scent, is celebrated for its ability to reduce stress. It contains linalool, a compound that plays a crucial role in calming the nervous system. This interaction with neurotransmitters helps promote relaxation and reduce the physical symptoms of stress, like a racing heart or tense muscles.

On the other hand, Clary sage oil is noted for its mood-supporting properties. Its earthy, slightly sweet aroma can help balance emotions and alleviate feelings of sadness or unease. By influencing hormone levels, clary sage can stabilize mood swings and promote a sense of well-being.

The effects of these oils extend beyond their pleasant scents. The science behind their benefits lies in their ability to interact with neurotransmitters and hormones. Linalool, found in lavender, affects the production of serotonin, a neurotransmitter that regulates mood, sleep, and anxiety. By increasing serotonin levels, linalool can help foster a sense of calm and contentment. Clary sage contains linalyl acetate, a compound that enhances its calming effects. This compound works similarly to reduce stress and create a balanced emotional state. The intricate dance of these compounds within the brain creates a natural pathway to emotional support, offering relief without the side effects often found in synthetic treatments.

Incorporating these oils into your life can be both practical and soothing. For on-the-go relief, consider creating a personal inhaler. Add a few drops of lavender or clary sage oil to a cotton wick inside a small inhaler tube. This portable solution allows you to take a moment of calm wherever you are. The act of inhaling these oils can serve as a mini meditation, offering a brief escape from anxiety. Blending these oils into bath salts at home can create a luxurious, calming soak. Imagine relaxing in warm water infused with the calming scents of lavender and clary sage as the day's stresses dissolve with each breath. This practice soothes the mind and relaxes the body, creating a holistic experience of comfort and relaxation.

The power of these oils is not just anecdotal; real-life stories attest to their effectiveness. Take, for example, the experience of Sarah, a marketing executive who found herself overwhelmed by the demands of her job. Anxiety became a constant companion, affecting her sleep and overall well-being. After trying various methods, she turned to lavender oil, incorporating it into her nightly routine. Sarah found that diffusing lavender in her bedroom helped her unwind and sleep better. The gentle aroma signaled to her brain that it was time to relax, easing her into a restful state. Over time, she noticed a significant reduction in her anxiety levels, feeling more balanced and in control. This personal testimonial is just one example of how essential oils can make a meaningful difference in managing anxiety.

These oils offer a natural, accessible way to support emotional health. By integrating them into your daily routine, you can create moments of calm and balance that help manage anxiety and depression. Whether through inhalation or a soothing bath, these practices offer a gentle reminder of the natural support available to you.

## 10.4 USING ESSENTIAL OILS IN MEDITATION PRACTICES

Picture a quiet room, dimly lit, where the hustle of the outside world fades away. This is your sanctuary, a space meant for meditation and inner peace. Essential oils can transform this setting, enhancing your meditation practices by adding an aromatic layer that deepens relaxation. The power of scent is profound, and when specific oils are used, they can create an environment of tranquility that enhances your focus and mindfulness. By incorporating essential oils, you invite additional sensory experience into your practice, helping to center your thoughts and deepen your connection to the present moment.

Frankincense stands out for its grounding properties among the oils known for supporting mindfulness and inner peace. Its rich, earthy aroma is an anchor, connecting you to the spiritual and the divine. Historically used in religious ceremonies, frankincense is highly regarded for its capacity to calm the mind, encourage introspection, and enhance meditation. It's a scent that invites you to breathe deeply, quiet your thoughts, and find a sense of stillness within. Sandalwood, with its warm and woody fragrance, complements this experience by enhancing the depth of meditation. It encourages a state of heightened awareness, allowing you to delve deeper into reflection and self-discovery. These oils offer more than fragrance; they provide a pathway to a serene state of being.

Incorporating these oils into your meditation practice can be simple yet transformative. Applying essential oils to pulse points before meditating can enhance your experience by allowing their aromas to influence your senses as you subtly prepare for your practice. Applying these oils becomes a ritual, signaling your mind that it's time to focus inward. Diffusing calming blends during meditation sessions also enrich the experience. The continuous release of their scent creates an atmosphere that supports relaxation and introspection. As you breathe in the fragrant air, the aromatic compounds interact with your brain's limbic system, promoting a sense of calm and focus. This sensory engagement helps deepen your meditation, allowing you to remain present and centered.

Creating personal meditation rituals with essential oils encourages you to explore what resonates most with your practice. Consider journaling with essential oil-inspired prompts. As you meditate, let the aroma guide your reflections and jot down any insights or thoughts. This practice enhances your meditation and helps track your personal growth over time. Combining oils with breathing exercises can further improve your focus. As you inhale the scent of frankincense or sandalwood, synchronize your breath with the rhythm of your thoughts. This combination of scent and breath keeps you grounded, enhancing your connection to your inner self.

**Reflection Section: Designing Your Meditation Space**

Think about your meditation space. How can you incorporate essential oils to enhance your practice? Consider the scents that bring you peace and focus. Experiment with different oils, noting how each affects your meditation. Adjust your space to include these elements, creating an environment that supports relaxation and clarity.

As you enrich your meditation with essential oils, you cultivate a grounding and enlightening practice. These natural aromas provide a sensory anchor, guiding you through the complexities of meditation with ease and grace. Embrace the scents that resonate with you and let them lead you to a place of tranquility and insight. In meditation, Essential oils enhance the experience and deepen your connection to the practice. In the next chapter, we will explore another facet of well-being—how essential oils can support physical health, revealing their multifaceted role in our lives.

11

# SEASONAL AND OCCASIONAL USES

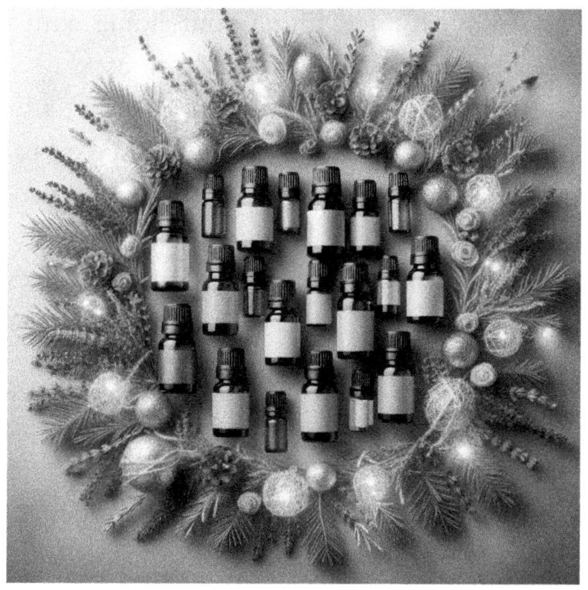

Each season brings its tapestry of memories and emotions as the year unfolds, often intertwined with the scents that fill the air. Imagine a crisp winter morning, where the aroma of cinnamon and pine greets you, reminiscent of holidays past. These scents are more than mere fragrances; they're gateways to the warmth and joy of festive times. Essential oils capture these aromas, infusing your home with the spirit of the season. They allow you to create a welcoming atmosphere for family and friends, turning any gathering into a celebration of the senses.

## 11.1 HOLIDAY SCENTS AND FESTIVE BLENDS

The holidays are a time when scents can transform a room, evoking memories of joyful gatherings and cozy evenings by the fire. Cinnamon oil is a staple in creating this ambiance. Its warm, spicy aroma evokes the scent of freshly baked cookies and mulled cider, filling your home with comfort and cheer. This oil can be used in various ways, such as adding a few drops to your diffuser or creating a delightful homemade potpourri. Pair it with pine needle oil to evoke a Christmas tree's fresh, evergreen scent. Pine needle oil is crisp and invigorating, its aroma reminiscent of a walk through a snow-dusted forest, grounding and refreshing all at once.

To capture the essence of holiday cheer in a bottle, consider crafting blends that encapsulate the season's spirit. The "Holiday Spice" blend combines clove, nutmeg, and orange essential oils. Clove's rich, warm notes pair perfectly with nutmeg's sweet spice, while a hint of orange adds a citrusy brightness that lifts the blend. This combination is perfect for diffusing in living areas or creating a festive atmosphere during holiday gatherings. Another delightful concoction is the "Winter Wonderland" blend. With fir, peppermint, and vanilla oils, this blend brings a sense of warmth and wonder.

Fir oil offers a resinous, woody base, while peppermint adds a refreshing minty coolness. Vanilla rounds it out with a soft, creamy finish reminiscent of snow-covered landscapes and winter joy.

Diffusers and candles are excellent tools for spreading these holiday scents throughout your home. Ultrasonic diffusers are particularly effective, creating a fine mist that disperses the oils evenly, ensuring a consistent aroma without overwhelming the senses. Make soy candles infused with your favorite holiday blends for a more intimate setting. Soy wax is clean-burning and retains scent, making it an ideal choice for homemade candles. Melt the wax, add essential oils, and pour into molds. These candles fill your space with warmth and light and serve as beautiful, personalized gifts.

Incorporating essential oils into your holiday decorations and gifts adds a personal touch that guests will remember. Infuse pinecones with your holiday blends by adding a few drops of oil, then place them in a decorative bowl or hang them on the tree. The result is a natural, aromatic decoration that enhances the festive atmosphere. Create personalized scented ornaments by crafting small sachets filled with fragrant rice or dried herbs, tied with a ribbon. These can be hung on the tree or given as thoughtful gifts to loved ones. Simple yet heartfelt gestures bring the magic of essential oils into the holiday season, enriching your home and gatherings with their timeless aromas.

## 11.2 WINTER WARMTH: COMFORTING BLENDS

As the days shorten and the air grows crisp, winter invites us to seek warmth and comfort indoors. Essential oils become allies, transforming spaces into cozy retreats. Ginger oil, with its spicy aroma, evokes warmth from within. It's refreshing scent heats the senses and brings a sense of vitality, perfect for warding off the winter chill. Cedarwood oil complements it beautifully, offering an earthy, grounding aroma that wraps you in a comforting embrace. Together, these oils create an environment where relaxation and contentment flourish.

Crafting the right blend can enhance this cocooning effect. The "Fireside Glow" blend merges cinnamon, cedarwood, and cardamom. Cinnamon's familiar warmth pairs seamlessly with the woody notes of cedarwood, while cardamom adds a touch of exotic spice reminiscent of mulled wine or spiced cider. This blend is ideal for diffusing in living spaces and inviting family and friends to gather and unwind. Alternatively, the "Warm Embrace" blend combines clove, vanilla, and sandalwood. Clove imparts its rich, spicy character, while vanilla adds a creamy sweetness. Sandalwood grounds the blend with its smooth, woody aroma, creating a scent that envelops you like a soft blanket.

Winter self-care routines benefit immensely from these warming oils. As the season often brings dryness, incorporating essential oils into body care can be soothing and restorative. Homemade body scrubs, enriched with oils like ginger and cedarwood, offer a gentle exfoliation that renews the skin. Combine sugar or salt with a carrier oil and your chosen essential oils for a scrub that invigorates both body and mind. Similarly, bath bombs infused with these oils create a spa-like experience at home. The warmth of the water releases the oils, filling the bathroom with a soothing aroma that relaxes tense muscles and rejuvenates the spirit.

Combined with these comforting aromas, mindfulness and relaxation practices gain a new depth. Evening meditation sessions, accompanied by the gentle diffusion of these blends, foster a sense of tranquility and introspection. Breathing in these scents can deepen your meditation, helping to center your thoughts and calm your mind. Warm compresses, scented with ginger or cedarwood, provide a simple yet effective way to unwind. Apply them to your shoulders or back, allowing the heat and aroma to ease tension. Enriched by essential oils, these practices offer a holistic approach to winter wellness, enhancing physical and emotional well-being.

## 11.3 SUMMER FRESHNESS: COOLING OILS

As the sun reaches its zenith and the days grow longer, we often seek reprieve from the summer heat. The shimmering haze and relentless sun can leave you yearning for a cool breeze. Thankfully, essential oils offer a natural solution to refresh and invigorate. Peppermint oil, known for its menthol content, produces a delightful cooling sensation on the skin. This oil is your summer ally, perfect for those sweltering afternoons when the air feels thick and still. With its lighter, more subdued aroma, Spearmint oil offers a gentle refreshment. Its subtlety makes it ideal for those who prefer a softer mint scent, providing a balm against the oppressive heat without overwhelming the senses.

Staying cool during summer isn't just about finding shade or a fan; it's about creating a personal oasis wherever you are. One effective method is crafting cooling body mists. Combining aloe vera gel with peppermint and spearmint oils creates a refreshing spray. Aloe vera provides soothing and hydrating benefits, while mint oils offer a refreshing cooling effect. Spritz this concoction on your skin for instant refreshment. Another simple yet effective way to cool down is adding a few drops of these oils to a foot bath. After a long day, a soak in cool water infused with mint oils can rejuvenate tired feet, leaving you feeling lighter and more at ease.

To capture the essence of summer, consider creating a blend that embodies freshness. The "Cool Breeze" blend, featuring eucalyptus, lime, and spearmint oils, is a perfect choice. Eucalyptus introduces a crisp, clean aroma, lime adds a zesty brightness, and spearmint ties it all together with a refreshing, minty note. This blend can be used in a diffuser to fill your space with a scent that evokes a pleasant, breezy summer day. For a more portable option, try a DIY cooling spray. Mix witch hazel with peppermint oil and a splash of water in a spray bottle. This simple yet effective spray can be a lifesaver, offering relief during outdoor activities or travel.

Keeping cool is crucial when you're on the move, whether it's a hike, picnic, or a day at the beach. Roll-on blends are convenient for on-the-go freshness. Combine a carrier oil like jojoba with peppermint essential oil in a roller bottle. This blend can be applied to the back of your neck or wrists whenever you need a quick cool-down. Adding a few drops of cooling oils to portable fans or cooling towels can amplify their effects. You'll enjoy an extended cooling sensation as the fan's breeze or the towel's fabric disperses the oils. These minor adjustments can transform your summer experience, making outdoor adventures more enjoyable even under the blazing sun.

## 11.4 ESSENTIAL OILS FOR SPECIAL OCCASIONS AND CELEBRATIONS

Imagine entering a wedding venue where a gentle floral aroma subtly enhances the romantic atmosphere. Essential oils can be pivotal in setting the mood for special occasions, transforming ordinary gatherings into unforgettable experiences. These natural scents can be the perfect finishing touch, adding depth and emotion to life's most cherished moments. Essential oils can elevate ceremonies and celebrations when incorporated thoughtfully, creating lasting memories for everyone involved. For instance, consider incorporating essential oils into wedding favors or ceremony rituals. A small vial of a calming blend can serve as a keepsake for guests, a fragrant reminder of the day. In the ceremony, oils like lavender or rose can be used to anoint the couple or as part of a unity ritual, symbolizing the merging of two lives. These small touches can make the occasion even more meaningful, embedding scent memories that guests will carry with them long after the day has passed.

Incorporating essential oils into party decorations and centerpieces is another creative avenue to explore. Imagine a table adorned with centerpieces that catch the eye and delight the senses with their aromas. Essential oils can be incorporated into floral arrangements or scent table linens, enhancing the atmosphere and making each table a focal point of sensory delight. For a more interactive experience, consider setting up personalized scent stations where guests can create their own aromatic blends. This activity entertains and leaves guests with a personalized memento of the occasion. Infusing table linens or napkins with essential oils offers a subtle yet impactful way to introduce fragrance into an event. A few drops of your chosen oil can be added to the rinse cycle when laundering linens, ensuring the scent is present but not overpowering. This technique can create a cohesive sensory experience, tying together the visual and olfactory elements of the event.

Creating celebratory blends tailored to the occasion can further enhance the atmosphere. The "Joyful Celebration" blend is perfect for a lively party or gathering. Combining lemon, ylang-ylang, and bergamot creates a bright, uplifting aroma that energizes and invigorates. Lemon brings a fresh, citrusy zest, ylang-ylang adds a floral sweetness, and bergamot introduces a hint of sophistication with its slightly spicy note. This blend can be diffused in shared spaces or used in personal scent stations, ensuring the party's energy remains high and spirits stay elevated. The "Romantic Evening" blend provides a deeper, more sensual aroma for intimate gatherings, such as anniversaries or romantic dinners. A combination of rose, jasmine, and patchouli creates a rich, luxurious scent. Rose, with its classic romantic appeal, pairs beautifully with jasmine's exotic sweetness, while patchouli adds an earthy depth that grounds the blend. This aromatic trio can be used in diffusers or candles, setting the stage for an evening filled with love and connection.

The versatility of essential oils allows for endless creativity in event planning. Experimenting with oils in DIY gift-making can result in unique, personalized favors that guests will treasure. Consider crafting custom blends that reflect the theme or mood of your event. For a garden party, a blend of geranium, spearmint, and lemon might capture the essence of a spring afternoon, while a beach-themed event could feature coconut, lime, and vanilla. These custom-made blends act as meaningful presents and carry the essence of the event's atmosphere, allowing the experience to linger even after its end. Encouraging personalization and experimentation with essential oils can lead to delightful discoveries and memorable experiences. By tailoring scents to specific events, you can create an atmosphere that resonates with guests, making each occasion memorable. As you explore the possibilities, remember that the power of scent lies in its ability to evoke emotion and memory, turning events into cherished moments.

12

# ADVANCED TECHNIQUES AND LESSER-KNOWN OILS

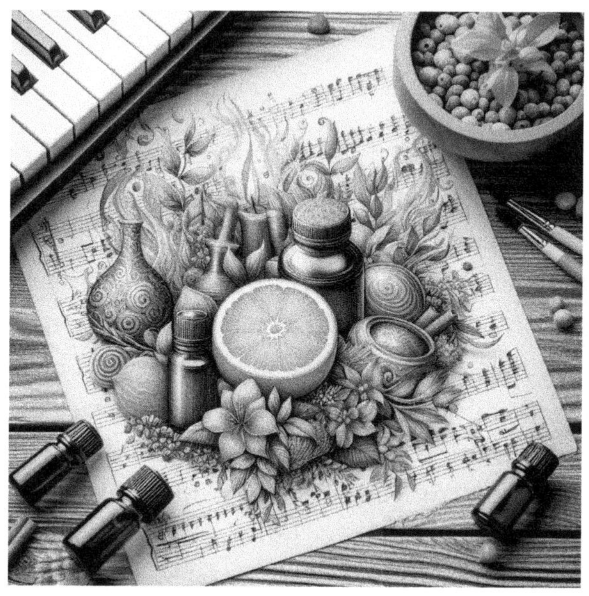

Imagine crafting a fragrance as personal as your fingerprint, which resonates with your essence and elevates your mood. This art of complex blending transforms essential oils into rich, multi-layered compositions. As you venture into advanced blending techniques, you explore the interplay of top, middle, and base notes. Each layer contributes a unique dimension to the blend, much like the components of a well-composed piece of music. Top notes, often citrus or light floral scents, provide an immediate impression; they are the first to greet your senses and typically evaporate quickly. Middle or heart notes emerge as the top notes fade, offering depth and character with scents like lavender or geranium. Base notes like sandalwood or patchouli linger the longest, grounding the blend with their rich, deep aromas. Understanding how these notes interact helps you create balanced, dynamic fragrances that evolve, captivating the senses with each unfolding layer.

## 12.1 CREATING AROMATIC HARMONY

The precision required in crafting such blends calls for specialized tools. Enter pipettes and graduated cylinders, which are essential for measuring exact quantities of oils. These tools ensure that each drop counts, allowing you to maintain consistency in your creations. Precision is critical, as even a single drop can alter the balance of a blend. Scent strips, meanwhile, become your canvas, enabling you to evaluate the aromatic outcome before committing to a final mixture. They allow you to explore different combinations, previewing how the oils interact once blended. This exploratory phase is crucial in achieving the desired aromatic profile, letting your creativity flow while maintaining control over the process.

Creating aromatic harmony is about more than just balance; it's about ensuring each component plays its role without overpowering the others. Modulating scent strength is one technique where you adjust the intensity of each note to achieve a harmonious blend. This might involve using fewer drops of a particularly potent oil or combining it with a milder counterpart to soften its impact. Longevity is another factor—how long you want the fragrance to last on the skin or in the air. By adjusting blend ratios, you can influence how quickly each note evaporates, creating a scent that lingers beautifully or fades gently, depending on your preference. These adjustments allow you to tailor each blend, ensuring it meets your aromatic goals while providing a satisfying sensory experience.

The journey of mastering complex blends is enriched by learning from successful examples. Consider a popular commercial blend that has made its mark in the fragrance world. Analysis reveals a sophisticated interplay of citrus top, floral middle, and woody base notes. This intricate layering creates a vibrant and enduring fragrance, appealing to various preferences. In the realm of therapeutic blends, the focus shifts to functional outcomes. A blend designed for stress relief might combine calming lavender with grounding frankincense and a hint of uplifting bergamot. The result is a soothing concoction that calms the mind and elevates the spirit, demonstrating how thoughtful blending can enhance well-being.

**Interactive Element: Create Your Signature Blend**

Try creating your signature scent to immerse yourself in the art of blending. Start by selecting a top, middle, and base note that resonates with you. Using pipettes, measure the exact drops of each oil onto a scent strip. Adjust the ratios until you achieve a harmonious balance. Record your successful blends, noting the oils and quantities used. This exercise not only hones your blending skills but also deepens your appreciation for the complexity and creativity of crafting personalized fragrances.

As you delve deeper into advanced blending, remember that each blend is a testament to your creativity and understanding of aromatics. It's a journey where intuition meets technique, resulting in scents that are as unique and multifaceted as you.

## 12.2 EXPLORING RARE AND EXOTIC ESSENTIAL OILS

The world of essential oils is vast and varied, offering unique properties and benefits. Some are less known yet hold remarkable qualities that can enhance your aromatic repertoire. Take agarwood, commonly known as oud, which boasts a deep, woody aroma often used in high-end perfumery and meditation practices. Its rich scent is calming and grounding, creating an atmosphere perfect for introspection or relaxation. Similarly, palo santo, often called "Holy Wood," is revered for its spiritual cleansing attributes. Traditionally used in South American rituals, its sweet, woody aroma is believed to purify and uplift, making it a popular choice for emotional and spiritual healing practices. These oils add depth to blends and offer profound sensory experiences that can enrich your daily rituals.

Ethical sourcing and sustainable practices become paramount as these rare oils gain popularity. The demand for exotic oils like agarwood and palo santo can lead to overharvesting, threatening their natural habitats and the communities that rely on them. Certification of sustainably harvested oils helps ensure that these oils are sourced responsibly. When purchasing, look for certifications that indicate sustainable practices, ensuring that your oils are not contributing to ecological harm. Overharvesting depletes natural resources and impacts indigenous communities traditionally managing and relying on these plants. Supporting brands prioritizing fair trade and sustainable harvesting practices is vital to preserving these precious oils for future generations.

The unique benefits of these lesser-known oils extend beyond their scents. Blue Tansy's distinctive blue hue is celebrated for its anti-inflammatory properties. It's often used in skincare to calm irritated skin and reduce redness. Meanwhile, Buddha Wood offers a different kind of tranquility. Its rare, earthy scent makes it an excellent companion for meditation and relaxation, helping center the mind and promote peace. These oils can be integrated into existing routines, offering new avenues for relaxation and healing. Whether you seek physical relief or a mental escape, these rare oils provide diverse applications that can enhance your well-being.

Given their potency and unique characteristics, it requires careful consideration to incorporate rare oils into your routine. Dilution is crucial, especially for high-potency oils like Blue Tansy and Palo Santo. A general guideline is to start with a 1% dilution, which equates to about six drops of essential oil per ounce of carrier oil. This ensures that the oils are safe for topical use and reduces the risk of skin irritation. Additionally, these oils can be blended with more common oils to create harmonious and balanced aromas. For instance, combining Blue Tansy with lavender can enhance its calming effects while adding a layer of floral sweetness. Understanding these oils' compatibility with others enhances their benefits and allows for creative expression in crafting personalized blends.

**Reflection Section: Responsible Sourcing and Sustainable Practices**

When choosing essential oils, it's crucial to contemplate the broader implications of your selections. The pursuit of rare and exotic oils while enriching your aromatic collection carries with it a responsibility to the environment and global communities. As these precious resources become more sought after, the risk of unsustainable harvesting practices grows, potentially leading to environmental degradation and socio-economic imbalances in producing regions. To mitigate these risks, it is imperative to support brands and suppliers committed to ethical sourcing and sustainability. This involves seeking out certifications that guarantee oils are harvested with ecological and social responsibility in mind. These certifications ensure that the plants are grown and collected in ways that do not harm their natural habitats, and that local communities benefit from the trade. Moreover, aligning your purchases with companies that prioritize the well-being of the planet reflects a commitment to not just personal health, but also to the health of our global ecosystem. This conscious consumerism helps maintain the balance of natural resources, ensuring that these potent oils can continue to be enjoyed by future generations.

Incorporating these considerations into your selection process does more than preserve rare essential oils; it upholds a philosophy of wellness that extends beyond the individual to encompass global environmental and societal well-being. This thoughtful approach to choosing essential oils reinforces the importance of sustainability in the ongoing journey towards holistic health.

## 12.3 CREATING POWERFUL OIL COMBOS

In aromatherapy, the combined effects refer to how certain oils, when mixed, can amplify or modify each other's effects. This dynamic interaction can transform a simple blend into a powerful tool for wellness. Take lavender and vetiver, for instance. Each is calming, but they create a particularly effective blend for promoting restful sleep. Lavender's floral notes soothe the mind, while vetiver's earthy aroma grounds the body, working to provide a more profound sense of relaxation. Similarly, combining tea tree and lemon oils enhances their antibacterial properties. Tea tree oil is a robust antimicrobial agent, and adding lemon enhances its effectiveness, resulting in a powerful combination suitable for cleaning or skin care.

Creating synergistic blends involves understanding the unique properties of each oil and how they can complement one another. For instance, make a blend that promotes respiratory health. A combination like the "Breathe Deep" blend, which includes eucalyptus, peppermint, and frankincense, can be particularly effective. Eucalyptus opens the airways, peppermint cools and refreshes, and frankincense adds a grounding element that enhances the overall experience.

This blend supports breathing and provides a soothing aroma that promotes relaxation. By experimenting with different combinations, you can tailor blends to suit your needs, whether boosting immunity, enhancing mood, or improving concentration.

Scientific research supports the use of synergistic blends for therapeutic purposes. Studies have shown that blending certain oils can enhance their efficacy, particularly in antimicrobial applications. For example, a study found that using a combination of antimicrobial oils increased their effectiveness against certain bacteria compared to using them individually. This suggests that combined oils enhance aroma and boost the therapeutic effects of the oils. Understanding these interactions allows you to create blends that are pleasing to the senses and offer tangible health benefits. By considering the properties of each oil, you can craft blends that meet your specific wellness goals, whether it's reducing stress, improving sleep, or supporting immune function.

As you experiment with creating your blends, keep a blending journal. This practice can be invaluable in tracking the effects of different combinations and refining your recipes. Note the oils used, their proportions, and your observations on their impact. This record helps you identify which blends work best for you and allows for efficiently replicating successful combinations. Additionally, consider adjusting your blends based on your personal aromatherapy goals. If you're improving focus, you might start with a rosemary base and add complementary oils like lemon or peppermint. The key is to be open to experimentation and willing to tweak your blends until you find the perfect combination.

The art of combining oils in aromatherapy opens a world of possibilities. By understanding how oils interact, you can create blends greater than the sum of their parts. Whether you want to enhance your health or enjoy the therapeutic benefits of essential oils, mastering oil blends can elevate your aromatherapy practice to new heights.

## 12.4 INTEGRATING ESSENTIAL OILS INTO HOLISTIC HEALTH PRACTICES

Picture yourself on a yoga mat, the gentle scent of lavender wafting through the air, guiding you into a deeper state of relaxation. This is where essential oils meet holistic health, enhancing practices like yoga and meditation. When integrated thoughtfully, oils can elevate your practice by engaging your senses and grounding your mind. During meditation, imagine adding a few drops of sandalwood or frankincense to your diffuser. These oils, known for their calming properties, can help deepen your focus and promote a tranquil state. Similarly, incorporating oils into yoga can enhance the experience through a calming lavender mist sprayed on your mat or a few drops of eucalyptus oil to invigorate your practice. The aromatic presence of these oils complements the physical and mental aspects of these practices, offering a multi-sensory experience that aligns with holistic health goals.

Beyond relaxation, essential oils can support dietary changes and overall wellness. Oils like ginger and lemon are renowned for their digestive benefits and can be used in culinary applications to enhance flavor while supporting digestion. A drop of lemon oil in your water can provide a refreshing taste while aiding your digestive system. Traditional medicine systems like Ayurveda, sandalwood, and frankincense have held significant roles. These oils are revered for their ability to balance the mind and body and are commonly used in rituals and healing practices. With its soothing aroma, sandalwood is often employed to calm the mind, while frankincense aids in spiritual and emotional well-being. Similarly, Traditional Chinese Medicine has long utilized ginger and clove oils for their warming properties and ability to support the digestive process. These historical uses underscore the profound connection between essential oils and holistic health, offering a time-tested approach to well-being.

Holistic practitioners often incorporate essential oils into therapies, illustrating their versatility and effectiveness. Naturopathy, which emphasizes the body's intrinsic ability to heal itself, frequently uses oils like tea tree or lavender for their antimicrobial and calming properties. Homeopathy, another holistic practice, may employ essential oils in remedies tailored to individual needs, further demonstrating adaptability. These practices highlight the potential of essential oils to complement various holistic approaches, providing additional tools for maintaining balance and health. By integrating these oils, practitioners can enhance their therapies, offering clients a comprehensive and personalized healing experience.

A personalized approach to integrating essential oils into your holistic health practices can be incredibly rewarding. Create a holistic health plan incorporating essential oils tailored to your needs and goals. Consider your daily routines and how oils might enhance them, whether using a refreshing citrus blend in the morning or a calming lavender scent at night. Incorporate oils into wellness rituals such as massages, baths, or even diffusing oils during quiet moments of reflection. This personalized approach allows you to explore how essential oils can support your well-being, fostering a deeper connection between mind, body, and spirit.

**Interactive Element: Create Your Holistic Health Plan**

Consider your wellness routine and identify areas where essential oils could enhance your practices. Choose oils that align with your personal goals, such as relaxation, focus, or energy. Develop a plan incorporating these oils into your daily life, from morning routines to bedtime rituals. Record your experiences and adjust your plan, ensuring it aligns with your evolving needs.

As we explore the integration of essential oils into holistic health practices, we see how these natural allies can play a significant role in our overall well-being. They offer a bridge between ancient wisdom and modern health practices, enhancing our lives with their versatile uses and profound effects. This exploration invites you to reflect on how these oils can become a part of your journey toward a balanced and healthy lifestyle.

# CONCLUSION

As we reach the end of this journey through the world of essential oils, let's reflect on the themes woven through each chapter of this book. We've explored how these natural wonders can enhance your well-being holistically. Essential oils offer more than just pleasant aromas; they provide accessible solutions for everyday challenges, from managing stress to improving sleep and supporting physical health.

Throughout the chapters, we've delved into various facets of essential oil use. We began by tracing their rich history and understanding their extraction methods to appreciate their purity and potency. In the chapter on safety, we highlighted the importance of responsible use, ensuring that you and your loved ones can enjoy the benefits of essential oils without risk. The stress relief, sleep enhancement, and muscle recovery chapters demonstrated practical applications, illustrating how these oils can seamlessly integrate into your daily routines.

We also explored the transformative potential of essential oils in breathing easier and cleaning the home naturally. These chapters underscored the environmental benefits of choosing natural solutions over synthetic alternatives, aligning with eco-friendly and sustainable living practices. Personal care and beauty, along with culinary uses, revealed the versatility of essential oils, transforming everyday tasks into opportunities for self-care and nourishment.

Safety and responsibility have been recurring themes, and for good reason. Using essential oils safely is paramount to unlocking their full potential. Throughout the book, we emphasized the need for proper dilution, patch testing, and understanding the oils' properties. By following these guidelines, you can confidently incorporate essential oils into your life, ensuring enjoyment and safety.

The benefits of natural solutions are profound. Essential oils offer a gentle yet powerful path to wellness. They support stress relief, enhance health, and promote eco-conscious living. You embrace a lifestyle that values simplicity, sustainability, and personal well-being by choosing essential oils.

One of this journey's most rewarding aspects is its empowerment. You're now equipped with knowledge and tools to personalize your use of essential oils. This book has aimed to inspire confidence in your ability to create a wellness routine that suits your unique needs. The recipes and techniques shared are just the beginning of what can be a lifelong exploration of natural health.

As you continue this exploration, keep experimenting and discovering new ways to incorporate essential oils into your life. The world of aromatherapy is vast and filled with possibilities. Whether crafting a new blend or trying a new application method, each step enhances your understanding and appreciation of these natural treasures.

I invite you to act starting today. Try out the recipes and techniques that resonate with you. Please make your own blends and adapt them to your preferences. Your journey with essential oils is personal and evolving, and I encourage you to embrace it fully.

Community is a powerful tool for growth and learning. Please share your experiences with others and learn from them. Join communities of individuals who are passionate about essential oils. Your insights and stories can inspire and guide others toward wellness.

I want to express my deepest gratitude for joining me on this journey. Your commitment to exploring natural solutions for health and wellness is truly inspiring. It has been an honor to share my passion with you, and I am excited to see how you will incorporate essential oils into your life.

I envision a future where essential oils are integral to your balanced, healthy lifestyle. Imagine a world where these oils contribute to your overall well-being and sustainability. This vision is possible and within reach as you continue exploring and embracing nature's power.

Thank you for your trust and curiosity. May your journey with essential oils bring you joy, wellness, and a deeper connection to the natural world.

# QUICK REFERENCE GUIDE

## A

- Acne: Apply tea tree oil diluted with a carrier oil to the affected area.
- Air Quality: Diffuse eucalyptus, tea tree, or lemon oil to purify the air and reduce airborne bacteria.
- Anxiety: Use lavender or chamomile oil in a diffuser or as a bath soak.
- Athlete's Foot: Apply tea tree or peppermint oil to the affected area.

## B

- Bloating: Massage peppermint oil onto the abdomen in a circular motion.
- Bruises: Apply helichrysum or lavender oil to the bruise.
- Breathe Better: Diffuse eucalyptus, peppermint, or rosemary oil to clear the airways and ease breathing.

## C

- Cough: Inhale eucalyptus or tea tree oil via a diffuser or steam inhalation.

- Cold Sores: Apply a drop of tea tree or peppermint oil to the sore.
- Cramps: Massage clary sage or lavender oil onto the affected area.
- Cold or Flu Comfort: Diffuse eucalyptus, peppermint, or tea tree oil to relieve congestion and soothe symptoms.

D

- Dandruff: Add tea tree or rosemary oil to your shampoo.
- Digestion: Use ginger or fennel oil massaged onto the stomach area.

E

- Earaches: Apply a mixture of lavender and tea tree oil around, but not inside, the ear.
- Energy Boost: Diffuse or inhale lemon or rosemary oil.

F

- Fatigue: Use basil or black pepper oil in a diffuser.
- Fever: Apply peppermint oil to the back of the neck and feet.
- Finger and Toe Nail Health: Apply tea tree or oregano oil to nails to combat fungal infections and promote strength.

G

- Grief: Diffuse rose or frankincense oil to support emotional healing.
- Gum Health: Rinse with a drop of myrrh or tea tree oil in water.

H

- Hair Growth: Massage rosemary or cedarwood oil into the scalp.
- Headaches: Apply peppermint or lavender oil to the temples and forehead.

I

- Insect Bites: Apply lavender or tea tree oil to the bite.
- Indigestion: Massage ginger or peppermint oil onto the stomach area.

J

- Jet Lag: Diffuse eucalyptus or peppermint oil to stay alert.
- Joint Pain: Apply a blend of eucalyptus and wintergreen oil to the affected area.

L

- Lack of Focus: Use rosemary or peppermint oil in a diffuser.

- Lice: Apply tea tree oil to the scalp and comb through the hair.

M

- Migraines: Use a mix of lavender and peppermint oil on the temples.
- Mosquito Bites: Dab lavender or tea tree oil on the bite.
- Muscle Aches: Massage in spearmint and peppermint oil.

N

- Nausea: Inhale ginger or peppermint oil.
- Nosebleeds: Apply a cold compress with a drop of lemon oil.

O

- Oily Skin: Add a drop of lemon or tea tree oil to your moisturizer.

P

- Pain Relief: Use peppermint or eucalyptus oil on the affected area.
- Psoriasis: Apply helichrysum or chamomile oil to the affected area.

R

- Rashes: Apply lavender or chamomile oil to the affected area.
- Restlessness: Diffuse lavender or sandalwood oil before bed.

S

- Stress: Diffuse or apply ylang-ylang or clary sage oil.
- Sunburn: Mix lavender or tea tree oil with aloe vera gel and apply to the skin.

T

- Tiredness: Diffuse or inhale peppermint or eucalyptus oil.
- Toothache: Apply clove oil to the affected tooth.

U

- Uplifting Mood: Diffuse orange or grapefruit oil.
- Urinary Tract Infections: Use tea tree or lavender oil in a sitz bath.

Y

- Yeast Infections: Apply tea tree oil diluted with a carrier oil to the affected area.
- Yoga Meditation: Use sandalwood or frankincense oil in a diffuser.

Z

- Zzzz (Sleep Issues): Diffuse lavender or cedarwood oil to promote restful sleep.

## POPULAR ESSENTIAL OILS

- **Lavender**: Stress relief, sleep aid, skincare
- **Peppermint**: Headache relief, digestion, energy boost
- **Tea Tree**: Acne treatment, antifungal, immune support
- **Eucalyptus**: Respiratory issues, decongestant, pain relief
- **Frankincense**: Anti-inflammatory, skin health, meditation
- **Lemon**: Cleaning, mood enhancement, digestion
- **Rose**: Skincare, mood improvement, anti-aging
- **Sandalwood**: Relaxation, skin care, aphrodisiac
- **Chamomile**: Sleep aid, skincare, anti-inflammatory
- **Bergamot**: Stress relief, skin care, mood enhancement
- **Cinnamon**: Warming, immune support, digestion
- **Clary Sage**: Hormone balance, menstrual relief, stress relief
- **Geranium**: Skin care, emotional balance, inflammation
- **Ginger**: Digestion, nausea relief, warming
- **Patchouli**: Skincare, grounding, stress relief
- **Myrrh**: Anti-inflammatory, wound healing, meditation

- **Ylang Ylang**: Skincare, mood enhancement, aphrodisiac
- **Rosemary**: Hair care, memory enhancement, circulation
- **Sage**: Respiratory support, memory enhancement, inflammation
- **Clove**: Pain relief, antiseptic, digestion
- **Juniper Berry**: Urinary tract health, detoxification, skincare

# ESSENTIAL OILS TERMINOLOGY

**Aromatherapy**: The practice of using essential oils extracted from plants to enhance physical, mental, and emotional well-being. It involves using various methods such as inhalation, topical application, and sometimes internal use under professional guidance.

**Base Note**: The element of an essential oil blend that evaporates the slowest and lasts the longest. Base notes provide depth and grounding to a blend and are typically derived from oils like cedarwood, patchouli, and sandalwood. They form the foundation of the aromatic profile.

**Carrier Oil**: A neutral, plant-based oil used to dilute essential oils before they are applied to the skin. Carrier oils, such as sweet almond, jojoba, coconut, and grapeseed oil, help to safely deliver the essential oils and prevent skin irritation while also providing their own therapeutic benefits.

**Cold Pressed**: A method of extracting essential oils, especially from citrus fruits, by mechanically pressing or crushing the plant material without the use of heat. This process preserves the natural properties and therapeutic benefits of the oils. Common cold-pressed oils include lemon, orange, and grapefruit.

**Diffuser**: A device that disperses essential oils into the air, creating a pleasant and therapeutic environment. Types of diffusers include ultrasonic diffusers (use water and ultrasonic waves), nebulizing diffusers (use air pressure to atomize the oil), and evaporative diffusers (use a fan to evaporate the oil).

**Dilution**: The process of mixing essential oils with carrier oils to reduce their concentration and ensure safe application on the skin. Dilution ratios vary depending on the oil and the intended use, with common ratios being 1-3% for adults and 0.5-1% for children or those with sensitive skin.

**Essential Oil**: A concentrated, volatile liquid extracted from various parts of plants, including leaves, flowers, stems, roots, and bark. Essential oils capture the plant's aromatic and therapeutic properties and are used for various applications in aromatherapy, skincare, and natural remedies.

**Evaporation**: The process by which essential oils release their fragrance into the air when exposed to the environment. This natural process allows the aromatic compounds of the oil to diffuse and be inhaled.

**Hydrosol**: The aromatic water that remains after the steam distillation of plant materials, also known as flower water. Hydrosols contain water-soluble parts of the plant and have a lighter scent than essential oils. They are gentle and can be used for skin care, facial toners, and room sprays.

**Middle Note**: The "heart" of an essential oil blend, which emerges after the initial top notes dissipate. Middle notes provide balance and are often the primary therapeutic effect of the blend. Common middle notes include lavender, geranium, and rosemary.

**Monoterpene**: A type of chemical compound found in many essential oils, characterized by its therapeutic properties, such as anti-inflammatory, antiseptic, and decongestant effects. Monoterpenes are often found in citrus oils and coniferous oils.

**Neat**: Using an essential oil undiluted, applied directly to the skin. While some oils can be used neat, diluting essential oils with a carrier oil is generally recommended to prevent skin irritation. Oils like lavender and tea tree are commonly used neat for minor skin issues.

**Oxidation**: The chemical process by which essential oils degrade when exposed to air, light, or heat. Oxidation can reduce the oil's therapeutic properties and may cause skin irritation. To prevent oxidation, essential oils should be stored in dark, airtight bottles in a cool, dark place.

**Patch Test**: A test to check for allergic reactions or skin sensitivities to an essential oil. To perform a patch test, apply a small amount of diluted essential oil to a small area of skin, such as the inner forearm, and observe for any adverse reactions over 24 hours.

**Photosensitivity**: A reaction caused by certain essential oils that increases the skin's sensitivity to sunlight, potentially leading to burns or irritation. Oils such as citrus oils (e.g., lemon, lime, bergamot) are known to cause photosensitivity and should be used with caution if skin is exposed to sunlight.

**Steam Distillation**: A common method of extracting essential oils, where steam passes through plant material to release essential oils, which are then condensed and collected. This method is widely used for oils extracted from flowers, leaves, and stems.

**Top Note**: The most volatile part of an essential oil blend, providing the initial impression and scent. Top notes are often light, fresh, and uplifting and are derived from oils like citrus fruits (lemon, orange) and herbs (peppermint, eucalyptus).

**Volatile**: Refers to the ability of essential oils to quickly evaporate and diffuse their aroma into the air. This property is what makes essential oils effective for aromatherapy and air purification.

**Wildcrafted**: Essential oils sourced from plants that grow wild in nature and are harvested sustainably without the use of chemicals or cultivation. Wildcrafted oils are often prized for their purity and potency, reflecting the natural conditions in which they grow.

# SUCCESS STORIES

1. **Emily's Focus Improvement**: Emily, a third grader struggling with attention issues, experienced significant side effects from prescribed medication. Her parents turned to essential oils and found that using specific blends helped Emily focus without altering her personality. They were thrilled to see their daughter's true self return.
2. **Michael's Family Wellness**: Michael used essential oils to provide a healthier lifestyle for his family. He was introduced to the oils by a friend and quickly saw the benefits, leading him to share his experience with others and positively impact his community.
3. **Linda's Skin Care Success**: Linda had persistent skin issues, including acne and dryness. She began incorporating essential oils like tea tree and frankincense into her skincare routine. Over time, she noticed a significant improvement in her skin's clarity and texture.

4. **Jessica's Digestive Health**: Jessica experienced frequent digestive discomfort and bloating. She began using ginger and peppermint essential oils by inhaling them or applying them topically to her abdomen. These natural remedies helped alleviate her symptoms and improved her overall digestive health.

# REFERENCES/SOURCES


*The History and Cultural Significance of Essential Oils* https://vriaroma.com/blog/118/the-history-and-cultural-significance-of-essential-oils:-from-ancient-times-to-modern-day?srsltid=AfmBOorJ3kr8UCvDXQmeYSVWuGXYiB2_LBkkh_L10N9UMFNuAWhNBxpL

*A Comprehensive Guide to Essential Oil Extraction Methods* https://www.newdirectionsaromatics.com/blog/articles/how-essential-oils-are-made.html

*Essential oils debunked: separating fact from myth* https://pubmed.ncbi.nlm.nih.gov/32463849/

*Pure vs Synthetic: The Truth about Essential Oils* https://aromahead.com/blog/pure-vs-synthetic-the-truth-about-essential-oils#:~

*The Complete Guide to Storing Essential Oils* https://www.matrixaromatherapy.com/post/the-complete-guide-to-storing-essential-oils-preserving-potency-and-prolonging-shelf-life?srsltid=AfmBOooQECBNUGoNLOP5kwkAjx7IVuoyFjZC0iZ-pbIBALfQdKw_CNoC

*Phototoxicity and Essential Oils* https://www.aromaweb.com/articles/phototoxicity-essential-oils.php

*Aromatherapy for Families: Safe Oils for Kids and Pets* https://www.myincensewaterfalls.com/blogs/aromatherapy/aromatherapy-for-families-safe-oils-for-kids-and-pets?srsltid=AfmBOop9E8q1OfpaTQxY6AGRq1xuP8gc7Ulrsaqb6d7mBpMCC_DuURo2

*Essential Oil Allergic Reaction - Healthline* https://www.healthline.com/health/essential-oil-allergic-reaction

*The effect of lavender on stress in individuals: A systematic ...* https://www.sciencedirect.com/science/article/pii/S0965229922000346

*10 Techniques for Reducing Stress Through Aromatherapy* https://breakingac.com/news/2024/oct/21/10-techniques-for-reducing-stress-through-aromatherapy/

*Essential Oils for Emotional Well-Being* https://www.aromaweb.com/essentialoils/essential-oils-for-emotional-well-being.php

*10 Essential Oil Diffuser Blends for Relaxation* https://www.aromaweb.com/recipes/relaxation-diffuser-recipes-blends-using-essential-oils.php

*7 of the best essential oils for sleep - MedicalNewsToday* https://www.medicalnewstoday.com/articles/essential-oils-for-sleep#:~

*Lavender and the Nervous System - PMC* https://pmc.ncbi.nlm.nih.gov/articles/PMC3612440/

*How to make your own dreamy sleep pillow spray - Pukka Herbs* https://www.pukkaherbs.com/uk/en/recipes/dreamy-sleep-pillow-spray

*Aromatherapy blend inhalation for better quality of life* https://tisserandinstitute.org/learn-more/aromatherapy-blend-better-sleep/

*Try 18 Essential Oils for Sore Muscles* https://www.healthline.com/health/fitness-exercise/essential-oils-for-sore-muscles

*10 Essential Oil Recipes for Pain Relief* https://www.labaroma.com/blog/10-essential-oil-recipes-for-pain-relief

*How to Use Essential Oils for Massage* https://www.bluetreearoma.com/blogs/a-life-of-aroma/how-to-use-essential-oils-for-massage?srsltid=AfmBOor7H3qnXCTEQog6JCVumf6jwJD7vWNUXe6aJBevC-Y8NeStNWow

*How To Make Pain Relieving Bath Salts With Essential Oils* https://soulfulsister.com/blogs/news/how-to-make-pain-relieving-bath-salts?srsltid=AfmBOooV82-d6SWk91zZOVB5jF-u8LOzG_ODWvjJR_hbhAwPXe7q4LBT

*Eucalyptus Information | Mount Sinai - New York* https://www.mountsinai.org/health-library/herb/eucalyptus#:~

*Top 7 essential oils for sinus congestion* https://www.medicalnewstoday.com/articles/324570

*10 Essential Oil Diffuser Recipes for Cough, Congestion ...* https://blog.whimsyandwellness.com/10-essential-oil-diffuser-recipes-for-cough-congestion-colds-flu-pdf-chart-you-can-print/

*How to Use Essential Oils Safely* https://tisserandinstitute.org/safety-guidelines/

*5 Benefits of Using Essential Oils for Green Cleaning* https://checklistmaids.com/5-benefits-use-essential-oils-cleaning-home/

*10 Best Homemade Air Freshener Recipes* https://www.theprairiehomestead.com/2013/06/homemade-air-fresheners.html

*Essential Oils That Kill Mold (And How to Use Them Safely)* https://www.mychemicalfreehouse.net/2023/03/essential-oils-that-kill-mold-and-how-to-use-them.html

*Homemade Non-Toxic Laundry Detergent with Essential Oils* - https://homemadeonourhomestead.com/effective-and-toxin-free-laundry-soap/

*Essential Oils in the Treatment of Various Types of Acne ...* https://pmc.ncbi.nlm.nih.gov/articles/PMC9824697/

*How to Create Your Own Essential Oil Blend - Natio* https://www.natio.com.au/blogs/discoveries/how-to-create-your-own-essential-oil-blend#:~

*9 Essential Oils for Hair Growth & Health - Healthline* https://www.healthline.com/health/essential-oils-for-hair-growth

*Easy DIY Body Butter and Lip Balm Recipe* https://parentingpatch.com/easy-diy-body-butter-lip-balm-recipe/

*How to Safely Use Food Grade Essential Oils in Your ...* https://labelcalc.com/food-grade-essential-oils-and-how-to-use-in-your-products/

*Essential Oil Dilution* https://aromatools.com/blogs/aromatools-essential-ideas/essential-oil-dilution

*Discover the World of Essential Oil Cocktails* https://bemoxe.com/blogs/news/world-of-essential-oil-cocktails?srsltid=AfmBOooRP2KYiBLhq_9lMhqbRyn_wSUruqXssKaORuigqPmF9v2PBM9B

*Cooking with Essential Oils - Savory Dishes* https://www.almarsa-gourmet.com/product-page/cooking-with-essential-oils-savory-dishes?srsltid=AfmBOoo58AIzmdOE5H-C9GevgnFjVqIvAky3Q5oxT5kUDefLlD3ZDrx_

*Cognition enhancing effect of rosemary (Rosmarinus ...* https://pmc.ncbi.nlm.nih.gov/articles/PMC8851910/

*Citrus Essential Oils in Aromatherapy: Therapeutic Effects ...* https://pmc.ncbi.nlm.nih.gov/articles/PMC9774566/

*Effects of lavender on anxiety: A systematic review and ...* https://pubmed.ncbi.nlm.nih.gov/31655395/

*Frankincense Magical Properties and Spiritual Healing* https://www.mdbiowellness.com/blogs/doctors-desk/frankincense-and-its-magical-properties

*10 Holiday Season Essential Oil Recipes - Diffuser Blends* https://www.labaroma.com/blog/10-holiday-season-essential-oil-recipes

*Top Cooling Essential Oils and Their Benefits* https://www.cliganic.com/blogs/the-essentials/top-cooling-essential-oils?srsltid=AfmBOor-eDpZ6PFKwOX_zM_dgDS_OQJI5COt1zTZpE7w7hN40indcLrg

*26+ Winter Essential Oils Blends For Diffuser And Skin* https://gyalabs.com/blogs/essential-oils/winter-essential-oils-blends-for-diffuser-and-skin?srsltid=AfmBOop0JWwlm3PjN9hYP_t3PyDjW6ouxqKIKcDRU2Tbrit7_8f23vab

*Scent-Sational Events: Using Aromatherapy for ...* https://thebelltoweron34th.com/blog/scents-of-occasion-using-aromatherapy-to-enhance-event-ambiance-and-memory/2024/10/3

*Therapeutic Blending of Essential Oils* https://www.aromaweb.com/articles/therapeutic-blending-essential-oils-guide-tips.php

*Exploring Exotic Essential Oils: Uncommon Oils with ...* https://www.heavenlypureoils.com/post/exploring-exotic-essential-oils-uncommon-oils-with-remarkable-benefits

*Synergistic Antioxidant and Antibacterial Advantages of ...* https://pmc.ncbi.nlm.nih.gov/articles/PMC8466708/#:~

*The Role Of Therapeutic Essential Oils In Holistic Health ...* https://www.pleasanthillsanctuary.com/therapeutic-essential-oils/the-role-of-therapeutic-essential-oils-in-holistic-health-practices

Essential Oil | Aurora Soaps. https://www.aurorasoaps.co.za/product-page/essential-oil

Essential Oils for Stress Relief - NourishDoc. https://www.nourishdoc.com/webinars/essential-oils-for-stress-relief

The Science Behind Aromatherapy and Its Benefits | Mi Foca. https://mifoca.com/the-science-behind-aromatherapy-and-its-benefits/

What are best natural ingredients for healthy skin – Rosa Herbalcare. https://www.rosaherbalcare.com/blogs/herbal-ingredients-for-hair-and-skin/what-are-best-natural-ingredients-for-healthy-skin

Essential Oils: Nature's Aromatic Extracts for Health and Wellness. https://www.graygroupintl.com/blog/essential-oils

Essential Oils for Hair & Skin. https://www.tonicessentials.com/post/essential-oils-for-hair-skin

Perfume Main Accords - The Ultimate Guide. https://perfumeson.com/perfume-main-accords-the-ultimate-guide

www.ingramcontent.com/pod-product-compliance
Ingram Content Group UK Ltd.
Pitfield, Milton Keynes, MK11 3LW, UK
UKHW021911190726
13853UKWH00002B/627